TALKING TOGETHER ABOUT LOVE & SEXUALITY

MILDRED TENGBOM

BETHANY HOUSE PUBLISHERS
MINNEAPOLIS, MINNESOTA 55438
A Division of Bethany Fellowship, Inc.

ACKNOWLEDGMENTS

My thanks to the young people who talked freely with me. Also to counselors of group homes, parents, the ethics professor of a Christian college and a gynecologist/obstetrician who kindly read the manuscript, critiqued it and offered many helpful suggestions.

Illustrations by Kent Vanderwaal

Copyright © 1985
Mildred Tengbom
All Rights Reserved

Published by Bethany House Publishers
A Division of Bethany Fellowship, Inc.
6820 Auto Club Road, Minneapolis, Minnesota 55438

Printed in the United States of America

Library of Congress Cataloging in Publication Data

Tengbom, Mildred.
   Talking together about love and sexuality.

   Includes bibliographical references.
   Summary: Introduces preteens and young teen-agers to various aspects of sexuality from a Christian perspective including the questions of contraceptives and premarital sex. Includes quizzes, exercises, and discussion questions.
   1. Sex—Religious aspects—Christianity—Juvenile literature.
2. Love—Religious aspects—Christianity—Juvenile literature.
3. Youth—Religious life. 4. Sex instruction for youth. [1. Sex instruction for youth. 2. Conduct of life. 3. Christian life.]
   I. Title.   II. Title: Talking together about love and sexuality.
BT708.T44   1985   241'.66   85-22837
ISBN 0-87123-804-7 (pbk)

THE AUTHOR

MILDRED TENGBOM was born in Minnesota, but has lived, not only in many parts of the U.S. and in Canada, but in various parts of the world as well. When she was 15 the Lord brought faith in Him alive in her and following that, little by little, God worked in her a willingness to turn her life over to Him. This involved relinquishing a dream of a writing career. Instead she went as a missionary to the borders of Nepal. On home leave she met and married Dr. Luverne C. Tengbom, and three years later, with two children, the family went to Tanzania, East Africa. After ten years of ministry there the family returned to the U.S. At that time she began to take courses in writing. She has had articles published in over 50 periodicals and is the author of 17 books. She also is a frequent speaker across the nation at conferences, retreats and seminars. In addition she has served on national boards of her church. Study and writing assignments have carried her to countries in Europe, Africa and the East. She is listed in *Personalities of the West and Midwest, Contemporary Authors* and *International Writers and Authors Who's Who*, and was one of 15 selected from 2,500 to attend a *Guideposts* Writers' Workshop. Her articles on the MIA/POW issue were incorporated into Congressional Records, and her book on Clara Maass has been placed in military libraries. Three of the four Tengbom children are in seminaries preparing for Christian vocations. With the children now out of the home the Tengboms have returned to missionary service, this time in Singapore.

BOOKS BY MILDRED TENGBOM

Is Your God Big Enough?
The Bonus Years
Table Prayers
Fill My Cup, Lord (with Dr. Luverne C. Tengbom)
Bible Readings for Families (with Dr. Luverne C. Tengbom)
No Greater Love: The Story of Clara Maass
Sometimes I Hurt
Help for Bereaved Parents
Help for Families of the Terminally Ill
Devotions for a New Mother
Especially for Mother
Mealtime Prayers
Why Waste Your Illness? Let God Use It for Growth
Does Anyone Care How I Feel?
I Wish I Felt Good All the Time
Does It Make Any Difference What I Do?
September Morning

FOREWORD

All too often books on sexuality by Christians have been billed as "frank and open discussions" but have exhibited considerable "Christian prissiness." Beating around the bush left their readers guessing at their meaning. Moral they were. Frank and open they were not.

Mildred Tengbom, happily, has committed no errors of obscurity or prissiness that I was able to discover. I cannot think of a sexual topic pertinent to the education of adolescents which has not been addressed completely, biblically and explicitly. Parents will learn a great deal too.

This is a book for adolescents, written to answer questions about sexual matters. Should one get involved in heavy petting? Are women's sexual needs as great as those of men? What, if anything, is wrong with masturbation? When are kids ready to get married? What qualities make a good marriage partner? Is oral sex sinful? What about living together before marriage? Why can't you have sex with the person you love and intend to marry? How does an IUD work? Can you prove you love someone by having sex? What is a condom? Can homosexuals change? Do girls masturbate as often as boys? What can you do to prevent being abused? Can venereal diseases be transmitted through oral sex? All these and many, many more such issues are addressed with frankness, sensitivity and lucidity.

The special merit of this book is the manner in which it was meant to be used: to help parents discuss sexual matters with their children. Without a resource like this book, discussions of sex usually will not take place at all in your family circle, or they will be kept at a superficial level, even if both parents and children have the best of intentions.

Parents, are you embarrassed about discussing sex with your children? Alas, I was during those years when our children were discovering their sexuality. My wife, however, was not.

For that reason the subject was an open one, in spite of my irrational anxiety about the entire issue in the presence of my offspring. Nevertheless, we did not approach sexual discussion systematically. But I believe that had we had Tengbom's book then, we could have done a much better job. As it was, our children received most of their technical knowledge of sex from the schools they attended. It would have been better had they acquired all their sexual instruction at home.

Let me urge you to get started in your own home—not merely reading this book, not merely handing it to your children to read, or if you are a teenager, not merely reading it yourself. Share it with one another as a family, as it was meant to be used. God will bless the household in which the Lordship of Christ is acknowledged also in the area of sexuality.

William Backus
Author of *Telling Yourself the Truth*

CONTENTS

Foreword   5
An Open Letter to Parents   9
1 / Who Says It's Easy to Be an Adolescent?   15
2 / How Much Do You Know About Our Wonderful,
    Incredible Bodies?   18
3 / Every Twenty-eight Days   31
4 / How Do Babies Come to Be?   39
5 / Have You Caught the Mystery and the Wonder?   57
6 / When Should I Start Dating? And How Will I Know
    When I'm in Love?   63
7 / Why Wait Until Marriage to Have Sex?   74
8 / When Will I Be Ready to Get Married?   99
9 / Contraceptives: Blessing or Disguised Disaster? 113
10 / The "Love Bug's" Dangerous Bite 134
11 / Questions and Answers on Tough Subjects 142
12 / How Can I Talk with My Parents About These
    Things? 153
13 / Years Later 156

AN OPEN LETTER TO PARENTS

Dear Parents:

You love your kids. More than anything else you hope they "turn out all right."

Now they're almost in high school—or already there. You tremble a little and wonder if you'll be equal to the years ahead. How will you know when to de-parent and when to continue to parent? How strict should you be? How many rules should you enforce? "If I just love my kids and trust them," you ask, "won't they turn out all right?"

Maybe. Maybe not.

One of the biggest mistakes you may make is not to talk with them about love and sex.

I can almost see you shrink. "That's not for me," you say. "Let the school or church take care of that."

Or you say, "I'll give them a book to read. But talk with them? How could I?"

Why not?

"Too embarrassing," you say, looking at the floor.

Why is it embarrassing? You don't have to reveal *your* sex life to your kids. In fact, you shouldn't. There's a place for privacy and respect.

But if we believe that when God said, "Very good!" after He created Adam and Eve, and included in that affirmation the sexual aspect of the two He had made, why are we so hesitant to talk about it? Sex isn't dirty. People can abuse it and make it dirty, even as they can abuse many other good and beautiful things. But sex essentially remains good—very good, in fact.

Now having written all this, I have a confession: I didn't find it easy either to talk with our four when they were adolescents. I felt awkward, just as you do. So I was glad for the help of several young couples at church who could relate well to our children. And my husband and I thank God for watching over and protecting our children.

But increasingly I have seen the need for *parents* to talk with their kids. If we leave our kids on their own, they're apt to come away with a lot of misinformation. Some of it could be downright dangerous. For kids are curious about sex, and they will find out about it whether it be from media, other kids, or adults.

Is there a family planning center in your area? What do you know about it? Are your kids going there? More kids go than parents realize. Because these centers promise confidentiality, these centers will never inform you, a parent, if your kids come for help.

What are kids hearing at these centers? What kind of "help" are they receiving? Dr. James H. Ford states:

> One of the chief objectives of the family planning counselor is to resolve the feelings of ambivalence and remove any feelings of guilt over illicit sexual activity on the part of young patients. The counselor tries to lead the young patient to accept his or her sexually-active lifestyle because one of the preconditions to effective contraception is a commitment to what the family planning industry calls "responsible sexuality"—that is, sex without babies. . . . Thus a direct result of the clinic counseling is to obviate, or at least to diminish the likelihood of a return to abstinence, and, in most cases, to increase the frequency of intercourse among clinic clients, and hence to increase their exposure to the risk of pregnancy.[1]

Do you know what your kids are reading about sex in books available in the school or public library? Consider, for example, these passages from a book for teens.

> Statistics, as well as our own experience, tells us that during your teenage years, your sex drive is probably at its strongest. *If you are not weighed down by inhibition and guilt* [author's italics], you are physically more potent sexually than at any other time in your whole life. Yet there are so many blocks to your achieving sexual fulfillment during your teen years, that the conflict presents a tremendous problem to you and to your society. It's a problem to you because of your driving needs versus your religious and moral beliefs.
>
> If you wish to follow your religious teachings, or those of your mother or father, then you may be confronted with some very uncomfortable feelings which must be handled in some

---

[1]*Linacre Quarterly,* May 1982.

way that is productive for you.

Self-satisfying caresses are not only harmless, they are desirable, satisfying, and safe. . . . Self-exploration and self-satisfaction can be very useful, and *is essential practice and preparation for heterosexual behavior.* (Author's italics.)

Usually, when you have very personal feelings and are puzzled about them, you want to talk to someone, but you don't know who. You think of asking Dad or Mom, but "they wouldn't understand." . . . They might, but you're afraid they'd put you down or discount your concern. Counselors at school are trained to listen, understand and help. . . . Give 'em a try sometime. TA groups are good too.[2]

Here is a quote from *How to Live Through Junior High School* (generally a good book) by Eric W. Johnson:

While there is much that can be done at home, I do not believe that home is the ideal place for all sex education. . . . It is important for the kids to have opportunities for discussions with their peers under the guidance of a knowledgeable, nonjudgmental adult. School (or perhaps institutions like the church or the "Y") is about the only place where such discussions can take place.

In the same book, Johnson discusses how questions about sex outside of marriage should be answered: "If your children ask you for your opinion, and you have one, give it, *but be sure it doesn't come out as an authoritarian viewpoint.*"[3] (Author's italics.)

In contrast to that opinion about authority, we need to hear the words of Karl Hertz, former Director of the Ecumenical Institute, Bossey, Switzerland, as he was addressing a group about the crisis of institutions today. Hertz commented: "The fundamental crisis of our day, not only in Western societies but globally, is that for large and important segments of the population the institutions (including the family) on which social order rests *have lost their authority.*" (Author's italics.)

The result? Trusting young people to arrive at right moral values, simply on the basis of logic, is dangerous if their faith in God and the authority of His Word, and in the authority of their parents have disappeared.

The question facing parents is this: Do you want your children's values and morals to be determined by the media, other

---

[2]Alvyn M. Freed, Ph.D., *T.A. for Teens* (Sacramento, Calif.: Jalmar Press Inc., 1976).

[3]Eric W. Johnson, *How to Live Through Junior High School* (Philadelphia: Lippincott, 1975).

kids, counselors in family planning centers and school teachers? If you don't, you'll need to start talking with your children.

It should encourage you to know that a recent survey among young teens revealed that sex is the subject they most want to discuss with their parents. When these teens were asked also to name the traits they considered most desirable in parents, they listed, far above others, "understanding." Surprisingly, love was not mentioned, possibly because young people tend to take love from their parents for granted.

But for those of us who say and hope that "just loving our kids will see them through," that answer from the kids should catch our attention. They want to talk with us about sex. And they want our understanding. If we are going to understand them, we will have to learn how to listen and how to communicate. Are we going to fail them?

A noted teen counselor has suggested that one of the best ways to start communication between parents and children is for both to read the same book and then discuss it. I hope this book will help you do just that. It is my prayerful, loving attempt to help meet your need.

As you use the book, remember that children mature at different rates. And children of different ages are interested in different things or have different views of the same thing. For example, Eric W. Johnson, in *How to Live Through Junior High School,* quotes these different answers to the question, "Would you like to go steady?"

Fifth grader: "In fifth grade???!!!"

Sixth grader: "It might be OK if there's no pawing and mauling."

Seventh grader: "I find I like a certain girl one week and a different one the next week, so how can I go steady?"

Eighth grader: "Yes. You can have a reputation and go to a lot more parties."

Ninth grader: "It's nice to have a steady girlfriend."

So you'll have to discern what is your child's level of maturity.

Talking about the physical, biological facts will be easiest if you start when the boys and girls are nine or ten—or younger. Besides, they need to know the facts by that age. Girls may become interested in dating and ask questions about behavior at an earlier age than boys.

Thinking ahead to marriage may seem out of sight for 13-

and 14-year-olds, but in these days of sexual permissiveness which can lead to pregnancies and premature teen-age marriages, parents need to begin talking with kids early about what it really means to be married. And all kids, from an early age on, need to know about social diseases (what a misnomer!) and contraceptives. Ignorance can be disastrous.

Knowing when to introduce each subject may not be easy. But children, by their remarks and questions, will let you know what they are thinking about and what information they need. Listen. Note their questions. Don't ever think it's too early. They are being bombarded on every side with sex and unbiblical attitudes and morals.

At the same time, try not to run ahead of them. Keep pace with each child's search for understanding. Many of us have heard the account of the mother who, in response to the question, "Where did I come from?" gave a detailed description of how babies come to be. Her child listened patiently and at the end said, "That was interesting, Mother, but all I wanted to know was where I came from. Beth says she came from New York."

How can you avoid such misunderstandings? One way to introduce a subject when a child or teen-ager asks a question is to turn around and ask him the question to find out what he is thinking. When you have identified the question or concern, this book may be useful to you in responding to that. Do not think you have to read this book through, starting from the beginning and going through to the end. Feel free to dip in here and there. Some subjects will be referred to more than once but in different sections. Our children are hearing the same messages over and over in the media and from their peers, so we do not need to avoid a little repetition either.

Remember also that, in one sense, education in sexuality has been taking place in your home for years. How you as husband and wife have expressed your love for each other, how you have treated each other, your children, and other males and females, will have spoken volumes to your children. This education is equally as important, perhaps even more important, than deliberate education. Both, however, are needed.

This book probably will be helpful if you and your children work out the little quizzes and exercises together and then discuss the answers together. If your children score higher than you on some exercises, hopefully you can chuckle and congratulate them. And remember, you still know more than they do about what love is and which values last.

And if, in the course of going through the book and talking with your child, uneasy memories of your own early years surface, memories that cause disquiet, discomfort and guilt, deal with those memories. Maybe the Holy Spirit will unearth buried incidents that need to be confessed so you can hear God's word of forgiveness pronounced.

Maybe, as you explore the subject with your sons and daughters, your own love and sex life will be enhanced and become more enjoyable and satisfying. Amen. Let it be so.

Finally, having done all you can to instruct your children, trust them. I remember the time one of ours came home at 4 a.m. I never made it a practice to sit up and wait for them to come home, but this time I awakened when the door opened. Horrified when I saw the time, I jumped in with my feet and mouth, not waiting for an explanation. As the hot words poured out, my beloved daughter broke down and began to sob.

Softened a little I asked, though still rather sharply, "What's wrong?"

The sobs continued.

Finally in short bursts the anguished words came out: "Mother, didn't you raise me?" She trusted my parenting. I didn't.

May God who loves us, who cares so much what happens to us and our loved ones, grant you wisdom and courage. May He give you and your children many intimate and meaningful conversations together.

Mildred Tengbom
Singapore

1 ❖ WHO SAYS IT'S EASY TO BE AN ADOLESCENT?

Meghan at Thirteen

Something's happening.

All of a sudden I've shot up, and I'm taller than all the boys in my class. How embarrassing!

I'm thrilled, though, that my breasts are beginning to fill out. I stand sideways and look in the mirror every morning to see if they've grown some more. But I'm worried because one breast is bigger than the other. I sure hope I don't end up lopsided. I stuff one side of my bra now to make up for the difference.

I hate the blackheads that have popped out around the corners of my nose and on my chin. How gross! I scrub my face every day, but they still appear.

I'm really wondering when my menstrual period will begin. I'm worried because all my friends have started. I wonder if I should see a doctor.

Peter at Thirteen

I can barely stand to look in the mirror these days. Has anybody ever had such a bad case of acne? How will any girl ever go for me?

Then to add to my misery, the medication the doctor prescribed prevents me from being in the sun. That means no more swimming, surfing or beach parties. That's real swift. But I don't think I'd care to be seen in swimming trunks now anyway—not with the acne on my shoulders and back. So basketball is out for me too. And I was good at it!

Plus, of all silly things, my breasts are filling out! Dumb things! A book I read said it's only temporary. I sure hope so!

Taking a shower with the other guys is embarrassing too. My penis is smaller than theirs and I hardly have any hair yet. The guys tease me. I hate it!

I've had to quit choir too. I can't sing because my voice ranges from a goofy squeak to a baritone.

And to top it all off, my girlfriend—at least the one I like to think of as my girlfriend—is taller than I am now. Adolescence! It's the pits! I hate it!

Feeling Confused

Adolescence is a topsy-turvy time.

It's exciting because all sorts of physical changes in our bodies are taking place. It's an anxious time because we wonder if we're developing fast enough or in the right way. It's a fun time because we get to participate in so many different things— away from our parents. But it's also kind of lonely sometimes, because other kids do some things we just can't feel right about doing. It's bewildering too because we don't want to talk with our parents, and we want to—both at the same time. It's a frustrating time when we have problems while other kids seem to be sailing right along. And it's a worrisome time because we have so many questions, and we hear so many tales, and we don't know what's myth and what's fact.

A doctor who works in a hospital emergency room said the other day that many 13- and 14-year-old girls come to the hospital with threatened miscarriages or other problems connected with pregnancy, but declare they don't understand how they could have gotten pregnant. That's really sad. For while adolescence presents us with exciting, fun times, it also ushers in a time of new and awesome responsibilities. The changes that are taking place in our bodies are preparing us for new relationships of love with those of the opposite sex. But, more soberly, those changes are preparing us also to become mothers and fathers.

But while our bodies mature so that, at a very young age we can "make babies," the other part of us, our personalities, our experience, and our ability to support and care for a family, has not reached the point of being ready or able to be responsible fathers and mothers.

Adolescence is therefore a time of waiting, of learning, of preparing. When we don't understand or accept this, but instead follow our emotions or try to act like grown-ups, we land in trouble.

We also land in trouble when we don't accurately understand our bodies and their powers of reproduction. So first of all, let's be sure we understand the different organs of our body and how they function.

2❖ HOW MUCH DO YOU KNOW ABOUT OUR WONDERFUL, INCREDIBLE BODIES?

> "People go abroad to wonder at the height of mountains, at the huge waves of the sea, at the long courses of the rivers, at the vast compass of the ocean, at the circular motion of the stars, and they pass themselves by without wondering."
> —Augustine

Our bodies are amazing! But how much do you actually know about them? Do you realize how complex their reproductive systems are? Do you understand what really happens in order to make a baby?

You've probably heard much information from other kids—sometimes as raw jokes during lunch hour or on the school bus. You can't, however, trust everything you hear. You therefore may not know as much as you think, and what you don't know *can* hurt you.

So, to help you know the truth about sex and reproduction, first test your knowledge on the next pages. After you've taken all the tests and corrected your errors, why not take the tests once again to be sure you've learned the right answers.

You may want to work out these exercises alone, or with your parents, or with a friend or two. Have fun!

What's Your Score?

(Answers on next page)

1. How many changes can you list that take place in a girl during her preteen and teen years?

    a. _____

    b. _____

    c. _____

    d. _____

    e. _____

    f. _____

2. How many changes can you list that take place in a boy when he enters puberty?

    a. _____

    b. _____

    c. _____

    d. _____

    e. _____

    f. _____

    g. _____

Answers to What's Your Score?

1. Changes that take place in a girl when she enters puberty:
   a. Her breasts begin to develop and attain a soft, rounded shape. They also may be sensitive and a little sore.
   b. Her menstrual periods begin.
   c. Her hips usually get rounder.
   d. Body fat gives a rounder, softer appearance to her body.
   e. Her voice gets slightly deeper and fuller.
   f. Hair begins to grow under her arms and in genital areas.

2. Changes that take place in a boy when he enters puberty:
   a. Hair begins to grow under his arms.
   b. Hair begins to grow in his genital areas.
   c. Hair begins to grow on his face.
   d. There is a thickening of hair on his arms, legs and chest. Sometimes hair extends from the genital area up to the navel.
   e. His muscles get thicker.
   f. His voice gets deeper.
   g. His penis and scrotum get bigger.

Who's "normal"? You are!

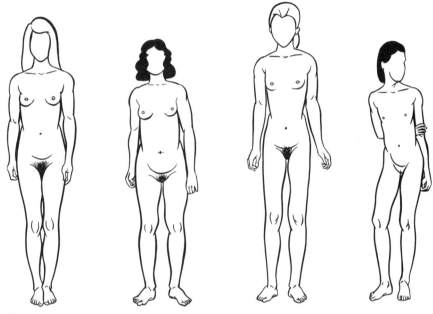

These four teen-age girls are all the same age.   Diagram A

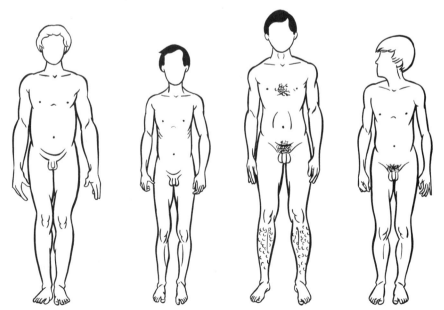

These four teen-age boys are all the same age.   Diagram B

It Pays to Know Words

Select the correct answer. In some cases one or more answers might be correct. Answers will be found on the pages following this exercise.

1. A man's genital organ is called (a) a scrotum, (b) an anus, (c) a penis.

2. The word *puberty* comes from a Latin word meaning (a) grown-up, (b) adulthood, (c) groin, (d) body hair.

3. Hormones are (a) sex glands, (b) chemical products in the body, (c) messengers, (d) sexual feelings.

4. Estrogen is another name for (a) ovary, (b) a hormone, (c) the sperm cells of a man, (d) the energy needed to have sex.

5. The pituitary gland (a) produces hormones, (b) helps hair grow, (c) is like a computer, (d) transforms a girl into a woman.

6. Breasts (a) give a woman a nice shape, (b) provide milk for newborn babies, (c) give pleasant sensations when touched in the right way, (d) are meant more for beauty than anything else.

7. Labia refers to (a) the lips, (b) one part of the brain, (c) the outer pair of "lips" between a woman's legs, (d) the cavity where a baby grows.

8. The clitoris is (a) the tip of a man's penis, (b) the opening through which a woman urinates, (c) a sexual organ in a woman at the head of the labia, (d) the opening in a woman's body through which a baby is born.

9. The urethral opening is (a) the opening through which bowel movements are eliminated from the body, (b) the canal in the ear that lets sounds in, (c) the opening through which babies are born, (d) the opening through which urine passes.

10. The vagina is (a) the opening through which a baby is born, (b) the opening into which a man places his penis during sexual intercourse, (c) the opening to the throat leading to the voice box, (d) a woman who has not had intercourse.

11. The hymen is (a) a gland secreting hormones, (b) a membranous fold that surrounds the vaginal opening, (c) a homosexual person, (d) the triangular patch of hair on the front, lower part of a woman's body.

12. A nonmedical name for the uterus is (a) cervix, (b) vagina, (c) womb, (d) stomach.

13. The endometrium is (a) the lining of the stomach, (b) the period when a girl has menstrual flow, (c) the lining of the

uterus, (d) the mucous membrane where a fertilized ovum attaches itself and begins to grow into a baby.

14. The cervix is (a) the top part of the brain, (b) the round shape of a woman's breasts, (c) the opening to the uterus, (d) the muscular walls of the uterus.

15. The ovaries are (a) the fatty tissues on the outside of a woman's body between her legs, covering the entrance to her body, (b) the name of the eggs formed in the woman's body, (c) the feeling of relief a girl gets when her menstrual period is over, (d) the sex glands of a woman that produce hormones.

16. The scrotum is (a) the long sexual organ of a man shaped like a finger, (b) the itching that results from some venereal diseases, (c) the small bag that hangs below a man's penis, (d) the place where sperm cells are produced.

17. The epididymis is (a) when an epidemic of venereal disease breaks out, (b) the skin covering the penis, (c) the place where sperm cells are stored, (d) the place where sperm cells are produced.

18. Vas deferens means (a) the vast difference there is between men and women, (b) the difference there is between being a boy and a man, (c) the difference between being heterosexual and homosexual, (d) the tube through which sperm passes.

19. To ejaculate means (a) the noise of pleasure one might make while having intercourse, (b) the action by which sperm is released from a man's body, (c) the act of having a bowel movement, (d) urinating.

20. Vulva (a) is the name given to all the external female genital parts, (b) the motion or movement made during intercourse, (c) the opening through which waste products are passed from the body, (d) another name for lips.

Answers to It Pays to Know Words
You will want to refer to the illustrations at the end of this answer section.

1. (c). A man's genital organ is called a penis.

2. (a), (b), (c) and (d). The word *puberty* comes from a Latin word meaning grown-up, adulthood, groin, and body hair. Puberty refers to that time when the body of a boy or a girl changes so the body becomes capable of reproduction. With girls this period usually is identified by the beginning of the menstrual cycle, though sometimes pregnancy can occur before the menstrual cycle begins. Other changes also take place.

3. (b) and (c). Hormones are chemical products produced by the endocrine glands. They travel in the bloodstream, acting like messengers, bringing messages to other organs, tissues and glands to change in certain ways.

4. (b). Estrogen is a hormone secreted by the ovaries. Hormones help develop a girl's sexual organs. They also control the functioning of the mentrual cycle and the production of milk for a newborn baby.

5. (a), (c) and (d). The pituitary gland is sort of a master control. It sends signals via hormones to the ovaries to produce more hormones which, in turn, cause all the changes to take place that turn a girl into a woman. Why does this happen only when a girl becomes nine, ten years old or older? Because our Creator God planned for the pituitary gland to produce another special hormone that acts as a guard, preventing the other hormones from carrying messages to the ovaries until a girl is physically mature enough to bear a baby. The pituitary gland is about the size of a pea and is located deep within the head, below the brain and in the center of the head.

6. (a), (b) and (c). Breasts do give a woman a nice shape, they provide milk for newborn babies, and they give pleasant sensations when touched. In some cultures they are valued most for the milk which they can provide for babies.

7. (c). Labia is the name given to the fatty tissue shaped something like big lips between a woman's legs that cover the opening to her body.

8. (c). The clitoris is a sexual organ in a woman found at the head of the labia. The clitoris has many nerves and blood vessels, and when caressed in the right way it helps make sexual intercourse a very pleasurable, fun experience for a woman,

sometimes leading to an extreme height of pleasure called "orgasm." The clitoris is covered by a soft fold of skin. It does not have any openings nor does it play any part in childbirth. It is there solely for sexual pleasure.

9. (d). The urethral opening is the opening through which urine is eliminated from the body.

10. (a) and (b). The word *vagina* comes from a Latin word meaning "sheath," the case into which a soldier slips his sword after using it. The vagina is like a tube or a canal. A man slips his penis into this tube when he has sexual intercourse with a woman. When a baby is born, it travels down through the vagina and out of the mother's body. The vagina is muscular and can expand.

11. (b). The hymen is a membranous fold that surrounds the vaginal opening.

12. (c). Another name for the uterus is womb. The uterus is the organ, or sack, in which an unborn child develops. The uterus is about the size and shape of a pear. The uterine walls are muscular and can stretch so a baby, which sometimes weighs over 10 pounds, can develop inside. A uterus can stretch until it may be at least 20 inches long.

13. (c) and (d). The endometrium is the soft, velvety lining inside the uterus. Many tiny blood vessels run through it. If no fertilized egg attaches itself to the lining, the lining breaks up and passes from the body in the form of blood during a woman's menstrual period. Then a fresh lining forms, all ready to give nourishment to any egg that might fasten itself to it.

14. (c). The cervix is the lower portion of and entrance to the uterus: it is the "stem" of the pear-shaped uterus. The opening of the cervix receives the sperm cells from the penis of the male.

15. (d). The ovaries are the sex glands of a woman that produce hormones. The ovaries also hold and release a woman's egg cells, called ovum.

16. (c). The scrotum is the small bag that hangs below a man's penis. The two testicles where the sperm cells are produced lie inside the scrotum.

17. (c). After the sperm cells are produced in the testicles, they pass into a strange-looking chamber called the epididymis to mature. The epididymis really is a tiny, thin tube about 20 feet long, but it has been kinked and curled up so as it lies next to the testicle it appears only about two inches long.

18. (d). After being stored for a while in the epididymis, the sperm passes up a 17-inch-long tube called the vas deferens on a journey to another small bag called the seminal vesicle where some of the sperm are stored. Normally a man has two testicles, two epididymides and two vas deferentia.

19. (b). The word ejaculate comes from a Latin word meaning to shoot out, to hurl, or throw out. When a man becomes sexually excited, the muscles in the genital area contract, causing the sperm or semen to shoot out. As this occurs, a system of valves shuts off the urine so none can enter the woman's body through the man's urethra.

20. (a). Vulva is the name given to all the external genital parts of a woman.

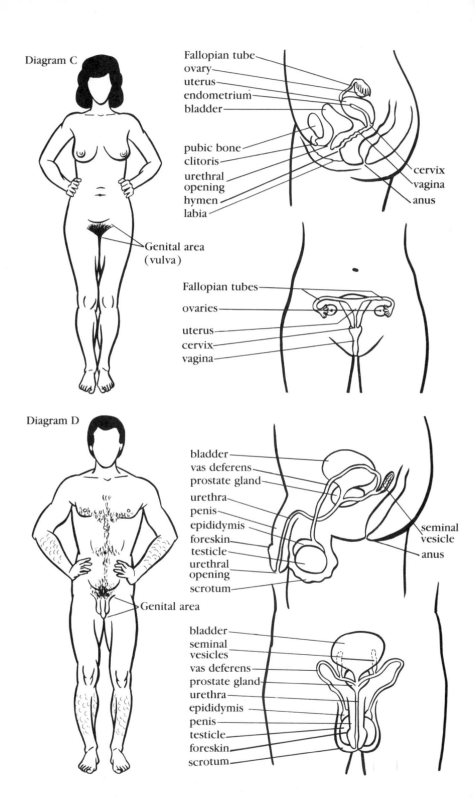

Diagram C

Fallopian tube
ovary
uterus
endometrium
bladder

pubic bone
clitoris
urethral opening
hymen
labia

cervix
vagina
anus

Genital area (vulva)

Fallopian tubes
ovaries
uterus
cervix
vagina

Diagram D

bladder
vas deferens
prostate gland
urethra
penis
epididymis
foreskin
testicle
urethral opening
scrotum

seminal vesicle
anus

Genital area

bladder
seminal vesicles
vas deferens
prostate gland
urethra
epididymis
penis
testicle
foreskin
scrotum

Review

Let's take a moment to review briefly, but in orderly fashion, what we've learned so far. How did you score on the quizzes? Better than your parents? Did you learn anything new?

About age nine or ten our bodies begin changing to prepare us to become parents. We won't be ready to actually be parents for a long, long time, but our bodies begin the process early. This period of growth and change is called *puberty*.

A tiny organ called the *pituitary gland*, about the size of a bean, hidden away in the center of the brain, starts the process. The chemical messengers it sends out are called *hormones*. The hormones chase through our bodies causing all kinds of changes.

Some of the same changes happen to both boys and girls. Skin becomes oilier. If the pores fill up with oil and the oil hardens, pimples or blackheads erupt. If the condition gets bad it is called acne. Washing the face regularly and avoiding fatty foods may help. Everybody hates pimples. In fact, in a survey teen-agers complained more about skin problems than anything else. Doctors, specializing in skin problems, often can advise on best treatment. These doctors are called dermatologists.

Young adolescents often are tired. This surprises and may worry them because they've been so used to having lots of pep and energy. But during puberty our bodies are growing fast and are changing. This is hard work. Because of this we need extra sleep. Our bodies also need balanced meals. Getting enough vitamins, protein and minerals is especially important. If we've been junk food addicts, we'd better change or we'll be sorry.

Voices change too. This is more noticeable in boys than in girls. Boys' voices may vary from squeaks to deep bass notes. But girls' voices also change and become more like women's voices.

For both fellows and girls, hair begins to grow under the arms and in the pubic regions.

Changes in Girls' Bodies

Now let's talk more specifically about changes that take place in girls' bodies, how girls with plain bodies get—as one little girl expressed it—fancy bodies like their mothers.

A girl's body has the capability of performing a special function. A girl's body, when it matures, can produce and care for a human life until that life is ready to live on its own outside the mother's body.

The place where this happens is the *uterus* or *womb*. Look at Diagram C to see where the uterus is. It's about the size and shape of a pear, but situated in an upside-down position in a woman's body. The uterus is lined with a soft mucous membrane with hundreds of tiny blood vessels. This lining is called the *endometrium*. It provides a nesting place for the fertilized *ovum* (an egg) and also provides food.

A canal, an elastic-like tunnel, leads from the outside of the woman's body to the uterus. This is called the *vagina*. The vagina is three to four inches long, but because it is muscular it can stretch. When it is not stretched the two walls lie against each other. The vagina receives the sperm cells needed to fertilize the ovum in the woman's body and transports them to the opening of the uterus called the *cervix*.

The ovum is stored and released from one of the two *ovaries*, one on each side of the body. Though each ovary is only about two inches by one inch in diameter, it contains thousands of egg cells.

The ovum makes its journey from the ovaries to the uterus via the *Fallopian tubes*.

The *hymen* is the membranous fold that surrounds the vaginal opening.

The outside genitalia of a woman are called *vulva*. Between a woman's legs are two pairs of "lips" called *labia*. One pair enfolds the other. The outer ones are fatty tissue and covered with hair.

The *clitoris* is covered with a soft fold of skin. It is very sensitive and responsive to touch.

A woman's body has three openings to the outside. The vaginal opening is where a man inserts his penis during intercourse. The *anus* is the opening through which waste products from the large intestine are passed. The *urethral* opening is to allow urine to pass from the body.

During puberty the shape of a girl's body changes noticeably. Fat redistributes itself, giving her body a softer, rounder shape. Hips enlarge. Breasts develop. Menstruation begins (we'll talk about this in the next chapter).

Changes in Boys' Bodies

Many changes also take place in a boy's body during puberty. In addition to having hair grow in the armpits and in the pubic regions, a boy often sees hair growing on his arms, legs, and chest, and a beard appears on his face. His features may become coarser. Changes in voice take place.

It may happen that different parts of his body grow at different rates. For example, feet or arms suddenly seem to become huge or long, causing clumsiness.

Changes take place in a boy's sexual organs too. Refer to Diagram D as you read.

A man's *penis* is about as long as a finger, but a little thicker, and houses a small tube from the bladder which runs down through the penis, to carry out urine. The other purpose of the penis is to carry the sperm from the man's body to the woman's. We'll talk more about that in a later chapter.

When a baby boy is born, the end of his penis is usually covered with a sheath of skin called the *foreskin*. This can be pushed back. Sometimes a doctor will remove the foreskin surgically soon after the boy is born. The operation is called *circumcision*.

Under the penis is a loose, wrinkled sac called the *scrotum*. Inside the scrotum are two oval-shaped glands about one and a half inches long called *testicles*. These are where the sperm are made. Behind each testicle is the *epididymis*, a coiled-up set of tiny tubes that store the sperm until they are mature.

The mature sperm cells travel through a long tube called the *vas deferens* to two small storage pouches called the *seminal vesicles*. These pouches lie at the back of the *prostate gland*. The prostate gland manufactures a thick, milky liquid called *semen* which helps the sperm travel down through the penis and into a woman's body when a man and woman have sexual intercourse. We'll talk more about this later.

3 ❖ EVERY TWENTY-EIGHT DAYS

Girls often develop earlier than boys. They grow in height so junior high girls are often taller than boys. You've probably noticed this. And when some girls are only ten years old (a very few are eight and nine), they begin to menstruate. We'll talk about that next. First test yourself to see what you know. Then the next section will answer questions often asked by girls.

True or False
(Answers on next page)

1. _____ Girls begin to grow rapidly at a younger age than boys.

2. _____ A girl's first menstrual period usually comes at the beginning of her growth spurt.

3. _____ After ovulation a girl can get pregnant any time until her next menstrual period begins.

4. _____ Girls can know when menstruation will begin for them by noting when their breasts begin to develop.

5. _____ It is possible for a girl to get pregnant even before she has her first menstrual period.

6. _____ If a girl has not begun her menstrual period by age 14, she should see a doctor.

7. _____ Some girls get depressed when they have their periods.

8. _____ Pubic hair begins to grow after a girl's menstrual periods have begun.

Answers to True or False

1. *True.* Girls generally begin their growth spurt about two years before boys do. During the time of a girl's greatest growth, her height may increase 2½ to 4½ inches a year. When girls are between 11 and 14 they usually are taller than boys.

2. *False.* Most often, though not always, a girl's menstrual period may come a year after her peak growth or three-fourths of her way through.

3. *False.* An unfertilized egg stays alive about 12 to 24 hours after entering the Fallopian tube. Then it breaks up and is absorbed into the body.

4. *True, to a degree.* On the average, though most people aren't exactly average, a girl's breasts begin to fill out about three or four years before her menstruation.

5. *True.* It has been known to happen that a girl has become pregnant even before her first menstrual period.

6. *False.* If a girl has not begun her menstrual period by age 14 she need not be concerned. Periods for girls begin anywhere from 9 to 17 years of age.

7. *True.* Some get weepy. Some, at least for the first months of menstruating, may have abdominal and back pain.

8. *False.* Pubic hair begins to grow about a year and a half before menstruation begins.

Questions Girls Ask

1. *What does the word menstruation mean?*

Menstruation comes from a Latin word *mensa* which means "month"—the old Roman calendar had 28 days in each month. A girl's menstrual period normally occurs about once every 28 days. Thus the word "menstruate" came into being.

2. *What actually happens during my menstrual period? Why do I bleed?*

The interior or the walls of your uterus are lined with a cushiony layer of blood and cell fragments. When a baby is going to grow inside a mother, this layer helps provide nourishment for the baby. When a baby is not growing, this layer breaks off and passes out of the uterus, down the vagina and outside the body. Because of the blood cells in this layer, the discharge looks like blood.

3. *How much blood will I lose?*

Usually only about five or six tablespoons.

4. *How many days will the bleeding last?*
Periods usually last from four to six days.

5. *When will I begin to have menstrual periods?*
That's hard to know. When did your mother and grand-mothers begin? That may affect it to some degree. Some girls begin when they are ten. A very few may start when they are only nine. Others may not start until they are 17. Usually about a year and a half before your periods begin your breasts will start to round out and hair will start to grow under your arms and in your pubic area.

The average age now for girls to begin their period is 12½. But don't misunderstand me. When I say "average" it doesn't mean you are abnormal if you don't start by then. Average simply means that's what the age averages out to be when you add up all the different ages at which girls begin their periods.

6. *For how many years will my menstrual periods continue?*
The time in life when menstrual periods stop is called men-opause. The average age of menopause is 51. There seems to be a family tendency with regard to age at time of menopause. If your mother had an early or late menopause, then you probably will have a tendency to follow that pattern.

7. *Which is better to use, tampons or pads or napkins?*
Your mother may have some good advice for you on this. Use that which is most comfortable for you and gives you the best protection. Some girls use both the first couple days.

8. *If I use napkins, how often will I need to change them?*
How often you will need to change your napkins, tampon or pad will depend on the amount of flow you have. Some days you may need to change every one or two hours; other days once or twice a day might be enough.

Used napkins should be wrapped in toilet paper and put in a disposal can, *never* down the toilet.

9. *How are tampons used?*
Complete instructions are included with every manufactur-er's tampon box. Simply follow the directions. If you think you're having problems, ask your mother or school nurse.

10. *Should I use two tampons on the first day to be sure?*
Never use more than one tampon at a time. Instead, you can

use a tampon and a napkin the first couple of days.

11. *Can I flush tampons down the toilet?*
Yes, you can flush both the tampons and the insertion tubes if the tubes are *cardboard*. Throw the plastic ones in a container.

12. *Won't the hymen prevent me from getting the tampon in?*
Tampons are small. Most girls are able to slip them past the hymen easily. Remember, the hymen doesn't cover the vaginal opening completely, and it is tissue and does stretch. Only a very few girls may feel discomfort when they try to insert a tampon. They should see a doctor who can help them.

13. *I started menstruating last year, but my periods don't come every 28 days as I read they would. Sometimes I wait two months. Once I waited four months. What's wrong with me?*
Probably nothing at all. Quite often it takes a girl from a year to two years before her periods occur at regular intervals. However, if you think you'd feel better about it, have your doctor check you. Chances are she'll reassure you that everything is okay.

14. *Why do I get such a heavy, bloated feeling in my abdomen during my period?*
Sometimes constipation can cause this feeling. Prevent this by eating fresh vegetables and fruit, whole grain breads, and cereal with bran. Drink lots of water—six or eight glasses a day at least. And exercise. All this should help. Reducing salt in your diet for six to eight days before your period begins may help. It's worth a try.

15. *Why do I perspire more during my period?*
Your sweat and oil glands are more active because of hormonal changes. Because you perspire more, it's important to give extra attention to keeping clean and using deodorant.

16. *Can I take showers and baths when I have my period?*
The first couple of days you may prefer to take a shower. However, if you wish, you may take a bath. When you take your bath don't have the water either too hot or cold. And change your tampon after your bath or shower.

17. *Why do I feel weepy when I get my menstrual period?*
A girl may feel depressed during her menstrual period because hormones can affect the nervous system. Hormones reg-

ulate the menstrual cycle and while they are doing this, they may at the same time change a girl's normal emotional balance.

18. *Why do I have cramps at the beginning of my period?*

Some doctors think some pain may be associated with a girl's attitude. If a girl resents having a period, or feels angry or upset about it, her pain may be greater.

Perhaps more often, however, the pain has a physical cause. Doctors think that tiny chemicals, such as hormones called prostaglandins, cause the muscles in the uterus to contract. If there are too many prostaglandins at work, the muscles of the uterus may contract so violently that a girl will feel pain. She may lie doubled up on her bed. If the pain is very bad, she may perspire or feel nauseated. Many girls feel some pain, either backaches or headaches or mild cramps, especially during their first years of their periods.

If the cramps are severe, see a doctor. One of the medications some doctors prescribe is a birth control pill. These pills prevent ovulation, and when ovulation does not take place, the prostaglandins are not produced. The menstrual period will continue to take place as usual, but without the cramps. Only a doctor, however, should prescribe these pills.

19. *Of all the medications in the drugstore, which one is the best for cramps?*

Aspirin is about as good as any, and probably the cheapest.

20. *Why does a girl skip periods?*

Occasionally a girl may skip a period. If she has gone through a traumatic experience such as having her parents divorce or having someone she loved die, she may skip a period. Even lesser tensions such as a test, a new living situation, or stress at work may cause irregular periods. If she has dieted severely and lost considerable weight suddenly, she may skip a period. If a girl has been following a strict vegetarian diet that hasn't included milk, eggs or meat, her body may not be getting enough protein or iron. Strenuous exercise, stress, excessive weight gain or rapid weight loss also can affect the frequency of menstrual periods. And, of course, if a girl has been engaging in sexual intercourse, there is the possibility that she is pregnant.

21. *When my first menstrual period begins, why does it start all of a sudden?*

It may appear that it starts suddenly, but it really doesn't.

It is part of a process that has been going on for a long time, a process by which a girl's body is being prepared to be capable of being a mother. Hormones control all the events of this process and this period.

22. *What are hormones?*

Hormones are chemical substances produced in glands. They travel to other organs of the body through the bloodstream, acting as messengers, telling other parts of the body how to respond or change. Hormones control the growth of boys and girls and the development of their sexual organs.

Reproductive hormones are produced in the ovaries of a woman, the testicles of a man, in the outer shell of the adrenal glands, and in the pituitary gland.

23. *Can I go swimming during my period?*

If you use tampons that will absorb your flow, why not? If you use napkins, stay out of pools and public bathing areas until your period is over.

24. *One of the girls at school says her mom won't let her go near the houseplants when she has her period because the plants will wilt and lose their leaves. Is this true?*

Absolutely not! There are all kinds of superstitious myths such as this floating around, claiming milk will sour, wine will taste like vinegar, etc. None of these myths are true. A girl's menstrual period is a perfectly normal, natural process, as normal as growing up, or as normal as digesting food or having to go to the bathroom.

25. *Can I play tennis on the first day of my period?*

Why not? Exercise is good for you. If you should find your bleeding gets excessively heavy after you've played (chances are it won't), taper off on your playing a little and take it easy for a day or two.

26. *I read that a girl has tiny eggs in her ovaries right from her birth, but they don't begin to develop or mature until she reaches puberty. Why is this so?*

During the first years a cluster of protective cells surround the eggs. These cells are called *follicles*, which comes from a Latin word meaning "shell" or "pod." A follicle is somewhat like a very tiny pod with a single pea inside it.

The egg or ovum is very important because it contains the

possibility for a new life. But the united egg and sperm can't make it on their own. They need help.

The hormonal system understands this, so it sends out a second hormone. This second hormone goes to work on the "pod" or follicle from which the egg has burst. The hormone changes the "pod" into a small clump of pinkish yellow tissue called corpus luteum.

The corpus luteum gets busy producing yet another hormone called progesterone. The word progesterone comes from a Latin word meaning "ahead of pregnancy," suggesting that this hormone will go ahead and get things ready in case a pregnancy takes place. What does the progesterone do? It makes the lining of the uterus soft, like a spongy mattress, so if the sperm and egg unite they will be able to snuggle down and find a nice, soft little bed there. The progesterone also orders the glands to secrete sugar and other nutrients to feed the new life. The placenta (the connecting organ between the baby's umbilical cord and the wall of the uterus) begins to produce the hormones, estrogen and progesterone, and these in turn send "messages" to the breast to develop and produce milk for the new life that has begun.

Wonderful, isn't it? If God has planned so carefully and minutely for bringing little babies into this world, shouldn't we be just as careful in not ruining His plan? He meant little babies to be born into homes where there is a mother and father who will love them and who are skilled and old enough to work and care for them in every way. It is true, of course, that sexual intercourse was meant not only to produce babies but also to bring pleasure and satisfaction to a husband and wife; but because pregnancy can happen whenever there is intercourse, intercourse should only be between a husband and wife, shouldn't it?

That was a long answer to your question, wasn't it?

27. *Is there any way a girl can know when ovulation takes place?*
Sometimes when the ripened or mature egg breaks free from its follicle or "pod," a little fluid escapes into the abdomen. If this happens, a woman may feel some twinges in her abdomen, and a very observant woman may be able to identify this as ovulation. Also, a very slight change in a woman's body temperature may take place, but it is so slight that most women would have trouble noticing it, unless they are daily recording

their temperature. Usually ovulation can be thought of as a quiet, hidden procedure. A girl or woman isn't really sure when it takes place.

28. *Will boys know when I'm menstruating? One of the girls at school says they can look in your eyes and tell. Should I wear dark glasses?*

If you did, don't you think they'd begin to wonder why you wore them only certain days each month? Don't worry. Boys usually don't know.

29. *Will boys' attitudes toward me change if they find out I've started to have periods?*

Maybe. Maybe not. They might know something about periods but not understand the process fully. They might think it is all very mysterious. They might treat you as though you could break—that is, they might be afraid to play rough and tumble with you anymore.

You might find that you really feel grown-up and suddenly the boys seem so young and you feel so old. You also might become more conscious of the fact that you're taller than many of them. Be patient. In two or three years things will level off.

Talk about the following questions with your mother, grandmother, older sister, aunt, schoolteacher or some woman you feel comfortable with and trust.

Some people tell girls that when they begin to menstruate, they become women.

Would you agree with this statement?

What do they probably mean?

What do you think it means to become a woman?

4 ❖ HOW DO BABIES COME TO BE?

"... to be able to create a human being who will breathe and move, walk and talk, love and hate, feel, think, work ... and know God! Oh, the wonder of it."
—*Devotions for New Mothers*
by Mildred Tengbom

Have you learned anything new as you've read? What seemed the most marvelous to you?

I was intrigued by a number of things—for example, the way the urine is shut off automatically when a man has intercourse. (What a relief for both husband and wife to know this!) And isn't it amazing that a gland the size of a pea, the pituitary gland, located deep in our heads, controls the hormone output of a girl, protecting her until she is old enough to bear a child? And imagine being able to curl up a 20-foot tube such as the epididymis so it can fit into a space about two inches long!

I marveled too at how carefully God has planned everything so all our body changes take place at the right time. There is a master plan behind it all, devised by a master Creator.

And all these body changes are planned so we can grow into people who can express love for another human through the means of sex. At the same time we are different from animals, who also experience sex, because we know sex, wonderful as it is, is only *one* expression of love. In fact, if other elements of a relationship aren't good, sex isn't good either.

I thought too of how humans are different from animals because humans know about death. That's one reason why understanding our bodies and the power we have over life and death is so tremendously important. We can create life. We also can destroy life. Awesome, isn't it?

Now examine that a little more in detail, okay? Do you really understand how to "grow a baby"? Come and find out, and get the facts straight.

True or False

(Answers on next page)

1. _____ A girl can get pregnant by kissing.

2. _____ A baby develops in the Fallopian tubes.

3. _____ If the sperm doesn't find an egg and unite with it, it passes out of the woman's body.

4. _____ When a little girl is born, she doesn't have any internal sex organs. They develop later.

5. _____ A boy is not born with sperm cells. They develop later.

6. _____ Even if a man can ejaculate 100 million sperm, he may be unable to father a child.

7. _____ The egg in a woman's body is about the size of a bird's egg.

8. _____ The male sperm is about 1/8 of an inch long.

9. _____ The sperm of the father determines the sex of the baby that is born.

10. _____ Human cells have 46 chromosomes, but the female ovum and the male sperm each have only 23.

Answers to True or False

1. *False.* A girl cannot get pregnant by kissing. The only way a girl can get pregnant is when sperm from a man's body unites with an egg in her body.

It happens this way: The man inserts his penis into the vagina of the woman. At the height of sexual excitement semen is ejaculated, or thrust out of the man's penis into the woman. The mucus, the slippery substance in a woman's vagina, grabs hold of the semen, and the sperm cells in the semen swim up into the uterus of the woman. But they don't stop there. Like little tadpoles they keep wriggling their tails till they reach the Fallopian tubes. If it is the right time in a girl's menstrual cycle, and an egg has been released and a sperm finds and unites with it, conception takes place, and a girl becomes pregnant.

2. *False.* A baby does not normally develop in the Fallopian tubes. After a sperm and an egg unite, the fertilized ovum (as the egg is referred to then) travels down the Fallopian tube to the uterus and attaches itself to the lining of the wall of the uterus and begins to develop. If a fertilized egg implants itself in the Fallopian tube (a "tubal pregnancy"), it must be surgically removed to prevent harm to the mother.

3. *False.* The unfertilized ovum passes out of the woman's body along with the mucous lining of the uterus in the form of the bleeding that takes place during a woman's menstrual period. The sperm cells simply disintegrate.

4. *False.* A girl is born with all her sex organs. There are even thousands of undeveloped eggs in her tiny ovaries. The

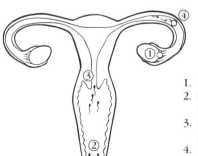

Diagram E

1. Egg is released from ovary.
2. Sperm enters uterus through vagina.
3. Sperm passes through the cervix and uterus.
4. Egg and sperm unite in Fallopian tube.

eggs start to develop and mature after a girl reaches puberty (from about nine years on, though it varies from girl to girl). Usually only one egg matures at a time. When the egg is ripe or mature and ready for conception, it is released. In the course of a woman's life about 400 or 500 eggs mature. Only a very few of these unite with sperm and develop into children.

5. *True.* A boy is not born with sperm cells. A man's body begins to produce sperm cells when a boy reaches puberty (at about 12 years). A man's body produces billions of sperm during the course of his life. When he ejaculates, there are from 200 to 500 million sperm cells in the semen, sometimes even a billion!

6. *True.* Even if a man can ejaculate 100 million sperm, he may be unable to father a child. Only one sperm is needed to unite with an egg for a baby to begin to grow, but the egg has a chemical coat that must be dissolved before the sperm can enter. How will the sperm solve this problem? Well, our Creator God planned it so all the sperm secrete an enzyme that is strong enough to dissolve the chemical coat. When the chemical coat is dissolved, a sperm can penetrate the egg. But it takes millions of sperm cells to produce enough enzyme to dissolve the chemical coat. If there are not enough sperm in a man's semen, there won't be enough enzyme to dissolve the chemical coat of the egg. So the sperm that finally succeeds in penetrating the egg has been dependent on the other sperm for his success; millions of sperm cells die in order that one sperm can enter the egg and produce a new life.

7. *False.* The egg in a woman's body is smaller than the period at the end of this sentence.

8. *False.* The male sperm is so small you can see it only through a microscope.

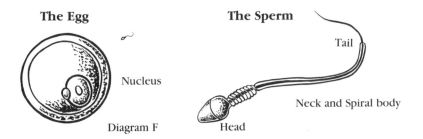

The Egg

Nucleus

Diagram F

The Sperm

Tail

Neck and Spiral body

Head

9. *True.* Every egg and sperm cell contains a sex chromosome. (A chromosome is a minute body that carries our genes, the things we inherit from our parents.) Egg cells always have female chromosomes referred to as X. But sperm may have either X (female) or Y (male) chromosomes. If a sperm with X chromosomes unites with an egg, you get two Xs and a girl is conceived. But if a sperm with a Y (male) chromosome unites with an X, you get XY and a boy is conceived. So it is the chromosome in the sperm of the man that determines the sex of the baby.

10. *True.* Human cells have 46 chromosomes, but the female ovum or egg and the male sperm have only 23 each. When the ovum and sperm unite, the new cell they create has 46 chromosomes, like all other human cells.

Multiple Choice

(Answers immediately follow this section)

Select the correct answer. In a few cases more than one definition will be correct.

1. The nucleus of an ovum is (a) the outer shell of the egg, (b) the path the fertilized egg takes when it travels from the Fallopian tubes to the uterus, (c) the center of the egg, (d) the gathering of sperm around an egg.

2. What percentage of inherited characteristics does a baby receive from his father? (a) 40%, (b) 60%, (c) 50%, (d) 55%.

3. Eggs are released from one of the ovaries of a woman (a) when a woman reaches orgasm during intercourse, (b) the first day of a woman's menstrual period, (c) about midway between a woman's menstrual periods, (d) all the time.

4. Ovulation means (a) an egg and sperm have united, (b) an egg is released from the ovaries, (c) an unfertilized egg is discarded in the menstrual flow.

5. Embryo is (a) the term given to the fertilized egg as it begins to grow, (b) the tail of the sperm, (c) the part of the egg and sperm that contains the genes, (d) the beginning of the menstrual cycle.

6. The umbilical cord is (a) the name given to the tail of the sperm, (b) the cord that fastens an embryo to the uterus so it won't fall out, (c) the "pipe" through which a fetus receives nourishment from the blood of the mother.

7. The placenta is (a) the act of placing the penis in the vagina, (b) the pancake-like organ of tissues and blood vessels that removes waste products from the growing fetus, (c) the flat organ in the uterus that allows nutrients to pass through its walls to nourish the growing fetus.

8. A fetus is (a) an embryo that is about two months old, (b) the medical term given before birth to a developing baby after organ development has taken place in the baby, (c) a fertilized egg, (d) tissue that, if left in the mother, will become a baby.

9. The amniotic sac is (a) the bag inside a man's scrotum where the sperm are stored, (b) the "bag of waters" in which the growing baby is protected, (c) the bag in the ovaries where the eggs are stored.

10. Labor pains are (a) the pains a mother takes to care for herself properly when she is pregnant, (b) the muscular con-

tractions of the uterus that push the baby out of the mother's body, (c) the pain a baby feels as it pushes its way out of the mother's body.

Answers to Multiple Choice

1. (c). The nucleus is the center part of an egg. It contains all the hereditary characteristics the mother will pass on to her baby: color of eyes and hair, size and shape of nose and body, degree of intelligence, musical aptitude, etc.

2. (c). A baby receives half (50%) his inherited characteristics from his father and half from his mother.

3. (c). A man's sperm is released during ejaculation, but the release of a woman's egg has nothing to do with sexual activity. The release of the egg is controlled by the pituitary gland in the head and by the ovaries.

4. (b). Ovulation occurs when a mature or ripened ovum or egg is released from a woman's ovaries. Most women don't know exactly when this happens. A very few women feel a twinge of pain. A few experience a little spotting (discharge from the vagina). But usually there is no indication at all.

5. (a). When the fertilized egg (that is, the egg after the sperm has penetrated it) moves down the Fallopian tube toward the uterus, it begins to divide. Some say it begins to look like a tiny mulberry. When it reaches the uterus it snuggles in close and clings to the lining. The lining has many tiny blood vessels to nourish the embryo. Then a little tube begins to grow out of the egg. This fastens itself to the wall of the uterus. This tube becomes like an intravenous tube that brings food and oxygen from the mother's blood to the embryo so it can grow. This tube also carries away waste products, such as carbon dioxide, from the growing embryo. In time this tube becomes longer and longer, and we know it as the umbilical cord.

6. (c). See comments above. The umbilical cord is joined to the baby's abdomen at a place we call the navel. The other end of the cord is attached to a flat organ made up of tissues and blood vessels. This organ is called the placenta.

7. (b) and (c). The placenta and the fetus lie close together. By osmosis nourishment passes from the mother's blood (in the placenta) to the growing baby. Also by osmosis waste products, such as carbon dioxide, pass to the placenta from the growing baby. The blood of the mother and the baby, however, never mix.

8. (a) and (b). After the first two months the embryo, which has developed so a head, arms, legs, fingers, toes and ears are all formed, is called a fetus. It is about an inch and an eighth long and lies all curled up. See the following diagram.

The Beginning of a Human Life.

Diagram G

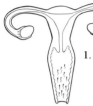

1. During intercourse, sperm cells are deposited in the vagina.

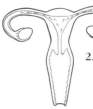

2. The sperm cells swim through the uterus and into the Fallopian tubes to fertilize the ovum.

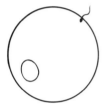 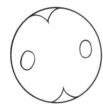 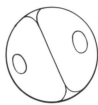

3. The fertilized ovum begins to divide repeatedly as the tiny embryo grows.

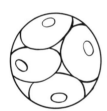 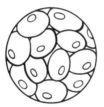 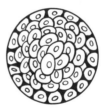

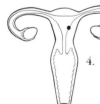

4. The embryo implants itself in the wall of the uterus.

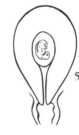

5. Within a month the human embryo is developing limbs and organs.

9. (b). God has provided a big, stretchable bag full of a fluid in which the growing baby can develop. This bag of fluid protects the baby from harm if a mother falls or is hit or injured. The fluid in the bag always stays at just the right temperature for the baby's comfort and growth.

10. (b). The baby doesn't work to get out. When the baby is

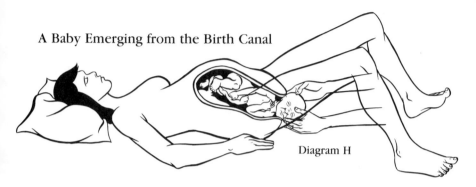

A Baby Emerging from the Birth Canal

Diagram H

about nine months old and ready to live in the outside world, the muscles of the uterus begin to contract and push the baby down. When the mother feels the muscles contract, she too pushes. This is called going into labor. Some pain will be experienced, though some women experience more than others. How much pain is experienced is determined by a number of things, such as the mother's physical condition, her attitude, her ability to tolerate pain. Usually a woman has more difficulty giving birth to her first baby than to subsequent babies. We do not know what the baby experiences as he is being born. But the birth of a healthy baby should be a wonderful moment for all, including the mother, father, doctor or midwife, nurses, relatives and friends.

True or False

(Answers immediately follow)

1. _____ A boy's penis enlarges and becomes stiff and erect only when the boy is sexually aroused.

2. _____ If a boy's penis has become erect because he looked at or thought of something sexual in nature, deliberately thinking about something else may cause the penis to become limp again.

3. _____ When a boy is born he is supplied with only a certain number of sperm cells, so he needs to be very careful how those sperm cells are expelled, saving them for the time when he wants to father children.

4. _____ Urine is passed from a man's body through a tube called the urethra which is in the penis.

5. _____ If a man has a big penis, he will have more sexual enjoyment during intercourse, and he will be able to bring more pleasure to the woman too.

6. _____ The scrotum is very sensitive not only to hard bumps and knocks but to temperature also.

7. _____ Male breasts, like female breasts, have sensitive areas which, if touched in the right way during intercourse between a husband and wife, can produce pleasurable feelings.

8. _____ If a man has enough actual sexual intercourse experiences to satisfy the needs of his body, he won't have "wet dreams" in which he loses sperm cells through ejaculation while he sleeps.

9. _____ If a girl has an unbroken hymen, it is proof that she is a virgin.

10. _____ The first time a girl has intercourse is always painful.

11. _____ A woman has one ovary that produces and releases one egg a month.

12. _____ As the egg journeys from the ovaries to the uterus, the egg passes through sort of a tunnel or tube called the Fallopian tube.

13. _____ A male hormone called testosterone tells a boy's body when it is time to begin to change and become like a man's body.

14. _____ A boy should begin to produce and ejaculate sperm cells at least by age 15 or he may never be able to do so.

15. _____ A man's body contains only male hormones, and

a woman's body contains only female hormones.

16. _____ Women have internal, hidden sex organs, but all of men's sex organs are on the outside.

Answers to True or False

1. *False.* Thinking about sex, looking at sex movies or read-ing sex stories may cause a penis to erect, but also if the bladder gets too full a penis may erect. If one is constipated and strains to have a bowel movement, the penis may erect. Even getting too cold, washing the penis, dreaming, or wearing too-tight clothes may cause the penis to erect. To experience the erection of a penis is a normal part of being a man.

2. *True.* Yes, some doctors say it is helpful to deliberately think about something else if one's penis has become erect be-cause of thinking sexual thoughts.

3. *False.* A healthy boy or man continues to produce thou-sands of sperm cells throughout his life.

4. *True.* The urethra serves double duty, as a channel for urine and as the outlet for semen during intercourse. The urine, of course, is shut off by a special system of valves so that only semen enters the woman's vagina. Well-planned, don't you think?

5. *False.* In fact, sexual enjoyment depends more on the brain than the size of genitals. When a penis becomes erect, smaller or larger penises tend to attain the same size. A relaxed penis, on the average, is about three inches long. When it be-comes stiff and erect it may be six inches long. It also gets a little wider.

6. *True.* When a man goes out in cold weather the scrotum shrinks up close to the body to keep warm. If a man takes a hot shower or bath, the scrotum hangs loosely, away from the body. In this way it protects the sperm inside the body that are very sensitive to heat. The scrotum is normally about one degree cooler than body temperature. The sperm could not survive at body temperature.

7. *True.* The nipple and the area around the nipple of a man's breast have many nerve endings that make them sensi-tive and responsive to touch.

8. *False.* Contraction of muscles that cause semen to shoot out while one sleeps is not an abnormal or wrong experience for a boy or man. Some say it occurs to release semen (or sperm cells) that has been piling up. Some say it happens in response to dreams. Having actual sexual intercourse does not prevent it nor does there seem to be any relation between the two. The ejaculation of semen during the night while one is asleep is a perfectly normal event.

9. *False.* The hymen may be broken by exercise, or it may stretch so much or so easily that it does not need to be broken.

10. *False.* In very rare cases the piercing of the hymen can be painful, but pain is not necessary. When a young woman is planning on getting married she should go to her doctor for an examination. The doctor can stretch the hymen if necessary. The doctor can teach the young woman how to do so herself.

11. *False.* A woman has two ovaries. They are oval-shaped like an egg and about two inches by one inch in size. They shelter thousands of eggs. Once a month, however, usually only one egg is released from one of the ovaries. Once in a while two eggs are released, and if sperm unite with both eggs, twins are born.

12. *True.* On the way from the ovary to the uterus, the egg passes through a sort of tunnel or tube called the Fallopian tube.

13. *True.* This hormone is produced in the testicles. This hormone also begins to produce sperm cells in a young boy.

14. *False.* A boy may begin to produce and ejaculate sperm cells anywhere from age 10 to ages 16, 17 or even later. Some boys develop more rapidly than others.

15. *False.* The bodies of both sexes contain some of each hormone, but in men male hormones are predominant, and in women the female hormones are predominant.

16. *True.* It would appear that one of the reasons for a man's sex organs being on the outside is that internal body heat could prevent the production of sperm. Sperm are produced in the scrotum, the little bag outside the body. The temperature of the scrotum is about one degree less than inside the body.

Questions Kids Ask

1. *I've read about a vacuum pump that will help my penis get longer. Would that be a good investment? I'm embarrassed when I take a shower because mine isn't as large as others.*

To invest in a vacuum pump such as described would be a waste of money. All of us have different body shapes and sizes. Even the size of penises will vary. The good news, though, is that when a man is sexually aroused and ready for intercourse, his penis, even though smaller when relaxed, will grow in size until it is almost the same size or the same length as the penis that, when in a relaxed state, is bigger than his. So don't worry.

The penis will fit into the vagina very nicely because the vagina is a muscular organ that stretches to accommodate the size.

2. *Is something wrong with me? When I have an erection, my penis isn't ramrod straight. It curves.*

Don't worry. It will assume the right shape when it penetrates the vagina.

3. *Is just putting a penis into a vagina all there is to sexual intercourse?*

Definitely not! Aside from the physical aspect, you need to understand the true meaning of intercourse. It is the most intimate way you can express love to a person. Through sex a husband can bring enjoyment, satisfaction, and feelings of security and being cared for to his wife; and the wife can bring the same to her husband. When a husband and wife engage in intercourse, their main concern always should be: How can I bring joy, pleasure, comfort, satisfaction and love to this one whom I love? Both the husband and wife do well to ask themselves this question.

Now when we talk about bringing joy to our mate, we know instantly that the physical act alone won't do it. We have to love that person and express that love in many different ways. Only then does intercourse have the meaning God meant it to have. Husbands and wives who quarrel, who don't talk much with each other, or who don't enjoy each other rarely can enjoy the sexual experience. Love is a many-sided thing.

And we need to stress again that intercourse is meant only for married people, for two people who covenant (promise) to love and be true to each other for the rest of their lives.

4. *Sometimes my penis gets erect when I don't want it to. And sometimes at night I wake up and I'm wet. What's happening? Is this wrong?*

Girls need to get used to their menstrual periods. Boys have their problems, too. Many of them feel embarrassed when their penises, sometimes suddenly and unexpectedly, become erect. They are afraid others will notice. Or they wake up at night and find a sticky, gooey wetness all over the sheets. They don't know what to do. They wonder if it will make the sheets smelly, or if it made any noise when it came out and if anyone heard it. Does it mean they have lost their moral purity? Some boys really worry a lot.

They don't need to worry. Most boys between 11 and 15 have this experience. It's another sign of growing up, of the body getting ready to father a child. What actually happens is that muscles contract, causing semen to spurt out. Semen, you will remember, contains sperm from the testes or testicles. Ordinarily this reaction, which is called orgasm or ejaculation, takes place when a man has intercourse. But if it happens at night while a boy is sleeping, it may be because of something he has dreamed. A boy does not need to feel he has sinned or done wrong if this happens. Instead, he can thank God his body is developing normally, and he can ask God to prepare him in every way for that momentous day when he will become a father.

5. *Why doesn't a baby drown in the fluid in the sac which surrounds him inside of his mother?*

An unborn baby does not drown because he is not dependent on his lungs for respiration. He does, however, make breathing movements while still in his mother's uterus. He also has amniotic fluid in his lungs. In fact, lung development is dependent on the presence of amniotic fluid.

6. *Does cutting the umbilical cord after birth hurt the baby?*

No, the baby doesn't feel it when the umbilical cord is cut.

7. *Can people who aren't married have babies?*

Yes, people who aren't married can have babies. Some people have sexual intercourse without being married. God's Word teaches us, however, that sexual intercourse is for married people only.

8. *If a wife is already pregnant, can she continue having intercourse with her husband or will she get pregnant with a second or third baby?*

If a wife is already pregnant, she may safely continue having intercourse with her husband until the baby is born, unless her doctor thinks there is a medical reason for not doing so. Hormones prevent a woman from getting pregnant again while she is pregnant.

9. *How can a person know the date a baby will be born?*

It is difficult to be absolutely sure of the date when a baby will be born. It takes from 270–280 days for a baby to grow and develop after conception has taken place. Usually a mother tries to remember the day her last menstrual period began. Then she adds seven days to that, counts back three months and adds a year; this gives a date fairly close to when the baby will be born, if all goes well.

10. *Why are some babies born with birth defects?*

There are many reasons why some babies are born with birth defects. Most of the time doctors don't know the exact cause of defects. Sometimes defects are passed from one generation to another. If a mother becomes ill with a certain disease while she is pregnant, the child may be deformed. For example, German or three-day measles (rubella) can cause deafness, blindness and mental defects. Certain blood differences between a father and mother can cause deformities. Some drugs cause defects and even some medicines a mother may take. Mothers using illegal, addictive drugs can give birth to babies suffering withdrawal symptoms. Cigarette smoking also affects babies.

11. *What happens when a baby is born feet first?*

A baby is born feet first only in about three percent of the cases. A doctor may turn the baby around inside the uterus before the baby is born, or may guide the baby safely through the birth canal. Such a birth is called a breech birth. Breech means "buttocks." Many breech births are delivered by Caesarean section.

12. *If a mother has to deliver her baby by an operation, will she have to have an operation every time after that when she gives birth to a baby?*

Surgery of this type is referred to as Caesarean section or procedure. Whether or not a mother will have to undergo surgery for just one or all of her babies depends on the reason for the original surgery, the type of uterine incision, the conditions of the next pregnancy, and the philosophy and training of the physician caring for her.

13. *When is a baby considered premature?*

A baby is considered premature if he has not remained long enough in the mother's uterus. An infant that is born three weeks before or two weeks after the due date is considered a full-term baby. Premature status is not dependent on the size of the baby, as some full-term babies may weigh less than five and one-half pounds if they have suffered from growth retardation in the mother's uterus.

14. *Aren't guys who are good at sports and who have strong, athletic bodies better lovers? Don't they have a stronger sex drive and don't they have stronger sperm to produce babies than guys who are frail and don't participate in sports?*

Body build makes no difference. Smaller, less physically robust men might be more considerate, tender, gentle, sensitive and understanding than those trained to be tough in competitive physical sports. Most women need gentle wooing in order to respond best, so men who are gentle, patient and understanding make the best lovers. And there is absolutely no difference in the sperm of either type of men or in the fertility of the sperm.

5 ❖ HAVE YOU CAUGHT THE MYSTERY AND THE WONDER?

Well, how did you do on those last tests? Learn anything new? I did.

Rethink, for a moment, all the steps by which a baby comes to be, and note the marvelous way God has planned for a sperm and egg to unite so a baby can be born.

As we know, men produce the sperm. We mentioned earlier that in order to protect the sperm which are very sensitive to heat, God arranged for them to be produced outside the man's body in a little sack (the scrotum). God also designed that sack so that in excessive heat, such as when a man takes a hot shower, the scrotum drops away from the body, but in cold weather it snuggles close to the body. The exact temperature must be maintained, and the body takes care of it automatically. The man never gives it a thought. Nor does the man give any thought to the billions of sperm being manufactured.

A boy's body doesn't begin to produce sperm until he reaches puberty, but a little girl is born with hundreds of tiny baby eggs in her ovaries. During the years the little girl is growing from being a baby to an active little girl, running around, jumping and playing, her body keeps watch over the little eggs so they won't mature. Deep within the girl's head is the pituitary gland. This gland is sort of a chief manager, sending out messengers (hormones) through the bloodstream to different glands of the body telling them when to do what.

The little girl isn't aware of any of this. She is carefree. She runs and plays and laughs and giggles, and her body is taking good care of her. But all the time she is growing and growing.

And as she takes care of a baby sister or brother or plays with dolls, she sometimes thinks of the day when she will be a mother.

When the girl gets to be nine or ten years old the pituitary gland begins to send messengers (hormones), telling her body to get ready for the marvelous adventure and experience of becoming a mother. The hormones run here and there through the bloodstream, telling various glands to get busy. Grow hair. Develop her breasts. Round out her hips. Give her whole body a soft, rounded shape.

Deep within the girl's body, in her uterus and ovaries, other changes begin to take place. It is time for the tiny eggs to begin to mature. The pituitary gland sends out a hormone to begin the work. Seven or eight days later it sends out a second hormone to help complete the work.

Each little egg lies protected in a "pod" or follicle. As the egg matures, it finally is ready to leave its follicle. It bursts free and floats into the Fallopian tube. If the egg could feel and talk, I would guess (wouldn't you?) that it would be excited. It would sense something new was about to happen but would wonder what it would be.

The destiny of those first eggs, however, will be different than the destiny of some eggs later on. The girl is still too young to be a responsible, tied-down mother. She isn't married yet. So because the girl is not married, and because she has no husband to plant sperm in her, the egg will pass out of the woman's body during the menstrual period.

At the same time the pituitary gland sent hormones to mature the tiny egg, it also sent hormones to prepare a nesting place for the egg in case it mated with a sperm. These hormones busied themselves in the uterus producing tiny blood cells and other nutritive substances.

The follicle of the egg changed its substance too, and began to produce another hormone, progesterone, which began to soften the walls of the uterus, making them cushiony and comfortable for the egg and sperm to nest in. But when the egg didn't mate with a sperm, all this preparation was not needed.

The first egg didn't find a mate, and maybe quite a few years will pass before an egg will mate with a sperm. All the time the girl's body is becoming better prepared to be a mother. Intellectually and emotionally, also, both girls and boys are being prepared to take up the responsibilities of being parents.

Finally the wedding day comes. Then in an act of love the

husband plants his sperm in his wife's vagina. Now a great drama begins.

What happens to the millions and millions of sperm the husband plants in his wife's vagina? They begin to swish their little tails back and forth, and they chase pell mell up the vagina and into the uterus. But they don't stop there. If it is the right time of the month, a little egg has burst out of its pod and is waiting for their arrival in the Fallopian tube. Somehow the sperm know the egg is there, so they jostle and push each other as they enter the tubes. When they find the egg they swarm around it.

Ever since the sperm entered the wife's body, they have been busy producing the special enzyme to dissolve the chemical coating around the egg. If there are enough sperm (hundreds of millions) to manufacture enough enzyme, the enzyme will dissolve the chemical coating. Can you image the excitement as the sperm swarm around the egg, pushing each other around, trying to find a spot where they can get in? If the egg could feel the coating around it beginning to soften, I'll bet it would be a little nervous, don't you think?

Finally one sperm thinks it sees a soft spot and dives at it with its little pointed nose; it dives with all its strength and succeeds! It enters the egg. The hole is quickly sealed off, and no more sperm can enter. The other sperm swim around, slowly die and then disintegrate.

What a marvel we see here! Only one egg a month matures and bursts from its follicle. The body takes care of this, and the woman doesn't think or do anything about it. Once in a while two eggs mature, sometimes as many as five, and then twins, triplets, quadruplets or quintuplets are born. But this is unusual. Suppose, however, the body wasn't dependable, that some months, instead of one egg, ten eggs matured at one time. What woman could survive giving birth to ten babies? But the body acts responsibly, and only one egg a month matures.

Maybe you are marveling, as I am, about the millions of sperm that never succeed in uniting with an egg. A lot of eggs are "wasted" too—about 400 to 500 eggs mature in the course of a woman's life. But of all these, how many become babies? One? Two? Six? Sometimes none.

"Why all this waste?" you may ask.

Actually, this "waste" demonstrates a principle of life. For example, if a flower goes to seed and those seeds drop to the ground, how many actually sprout and grow? Only a few. If you play the piano, how many hours must you practice before you can play a composition without mistakes and with feeling? Many. If you study for a test, you cram much information into your head—but how much do you actually use to answer the questions? Only some of it. For every good accomplishment in life, a lot of effort has been expended in one way or another that could appear to have been wasted.

In the same way you and I have come into being at the expense of millions of sperm which died in the attempt. If they had not sacrificed themselves, we would not be. If our mothers had not been willing to shelter us in their wombs and endure discomfort and pain, we would not be. And if Jesus had not been willing to give His life and die for us, the life we know now could not be an eternal life with God, even after death. Think of all the sacrifice that was made for each of us. We are very valuable!

And you and I are marvels. When an egg with 23 chromosomes unites with a sperm with 23 chromosomes, the two become a living cell, like all other cells in the body which have 46 chromosomes. The two incompletes become a whole.

Each sperm and egg contains a different "mix" of chromosomes. The chromosomes carry all the genetic characteristics that make you what you are: short or tall, slim or inclined to be chubby, dark-skinned or light-skinned, black-haired or blonde, happy-go-lucky or serious, musical or mechanical, etc. But think. If any other sperm than the one that united with the egg in your mother's body had united with the egg, you would be a different person. Isn't that awesome? Certainly God was watching over you even as you were being formed. The Psalmist believed it, so he wrote:

> You made all the delicate, inner parts of my body, and knit them together in my mother's womb. Thank you for making me so wonderfully complex! It is amazing to think about. Your workmanship is marvelous—and how well I know it. You were there while I was being formed in utter seclusion! You saw me before I was born and scheduled each day of my life before I began to breathe. Every day was recorded in your Book! How precious it is, Lord, to realize that you are thinking about me constantly! I can't even count how many times a day your thoughts turn towards me. And when I waken in the morning, you are still thinking of me! (Ps. 139:13–18, TLB)

But the marvels aren't over. We described earlier the process whereby, while the egg is ripening, the uterus is being prepared to be a cushiony, warm, protective, nourishing home for the mated sperm and egg. The united sperm and egg now swim down to the uterus and burrow into its wall. The egg grows a little tube that fastens itself to an organ called the placenta. Through this tube, the umbilical cord, the new developing baby being is fed and its waste products are carried away.

The body gears up now that a new life is being formed. The pituitary gland sends out orders via its messengers—hormones. No more eggs are to be matured until the baby is born. Menstruation must cease.

The mother's breasts must get ready to produce milk for the baby when he is born. The body is thinking way ahead, planning for that momentous hour about nine months away when the baby will be born.

But the greatest mystery of all is that although a husband and wife share in bringing a physical life into being, God steps in and breathes into that new life a soul. This new soul, however, later will be able to respond in love to God and others, but also will be able to turn its back on its Creator.

A soul is what really makes a person a person. To understand this we only need to look at a body after a person has died. Though we recognize the body, the person, as we knew him when he was living, just isn't there. Though all Christians don't exactly agree on what happens to the soul after death, we know that our souls are in God's care. Souls live on forever, and those who put their faith in Christ will one day find homes again in new bodies fashioned after Jesus' own resurrection body.

Now as we retrace the marvelous and detailed way God has planned for our body responsibly, faithfully and quietly to carry out its task of bringing a new life to birth, we should say to ourselves: "I want to be just as responsible and careful as God. Even as God has provided a warm, safe place for the baby to grow, so I must be sure that I, with a husband or wife, can provide a safe, secure, loving and warm home for our baby to grow. I will not play around with the reproductive part of my body by having sex before I am married. I will love my body and honor and respect its reproductive powers. I will show God that even as He has trusted me with the power to become a parent, He can trust me to use those powers only as He has planned that they should be used."

It won't be easy, however, to stick to that resolve when the pressure gets heavy. I'll bet you're already feeling the pressure in school to have sex, aren't you? Or if you haven't felt it yet, you will. Strangely, these days the ones who don't want to have sex until they are married are considered the odd ones, the nerds, the ones who are ridiculed.

So let's discuss in the next chapter how we can live up to our resolve to protect our wonderful sexuality until marriage.

6 ❖ WHEN SHOULD I START DATING? AND HOW WILL I KNOW WHEN I'M IN LOVE?

Questions Kids Ask

1. *I'm fourteen. My parents still have rules about how often I can date, what time I have to be home, etc. I think I'm old enough to make these decisions by myself. What can I do?*

Talk with your parents. Tell them how you feel. Explain why you feel as you do. Don't harangue or scold or yell at them, and don't tell them they don't understand. Just tell them your point of view. And at the end, tell them you love them.

Then ask your parents to tell you their point of view. Hopefully they'll do this calmly and won't yell at you either. Listen to them. That means trying to step into their shoes in order to see things from their point of view. After all, they are concerned for you. Don't be listening with half an ear while your brain is figuring out an answer to everything they say. After they have talked, get alone by yourself and think. Are there any points you think are negotiable? If there are, ask your parents if you can talk with them again.

Different parents create different rules for a number of different reasons. But usually teen-agers can be sure their parents love them and want only the best for them. If parents have rules, very often it's simply because they want to help and protect their sons or daughters until those kids are old enough, or responsible and trustworthy enough to live without rules. The most convincing argument you can give is to show, in every way you can, that you are responsible and trustworthy. If you act like an adult, your parents will treat you as an adult. If you don't, well . . .

2. *How can I really know what true love is?*

That's a difficult question but a good one to ask. It's difficult because especially when you're a teen-ager and just beginning to learn about love you often confuse love with infatuation—a "crush." Quite possibly you'll go through eight to a dozen cases of infatuation before you begin to really love someone. The question of what is true love is a good one to ask because marriages increasingly are lasting only a few years. Divorce always brings hurt and heartache, so you want to do everything you can to prevent it, don't you? Therefore it is wise to proceed slowly and cautiously in your relationships.

Here are some differences between infatuation, or having a crush, and true love. Thinking about them may help you understand what true love is.

Infatuation	*True love*
a. The person's physical appearance and dress are very important.	a. Physical appearance is not the most important. You might even find yourself loving someone who is quite the opposite in appearance from what your original "ideal" was.
b. You are most conscious of how this person excites you sexually.	b. You like to touch and be close to the person, but you also are just good friends and enjoy doing things together.
c. When you are together, you think about and spend a lot of time kissing and making out.	c. You enjoy doing things together such as playing tennis, etc. Showing affection is just part of your time together, though you always are courteous and respectful toward each other.
d. You can't see anything wrong in the other person.	d. The other person sometimes does things that annoy you, but you learn how to work out these problems.
e. You are afraid of being your true self lest the other person won't like you, so you pretend a lot.	e. You know you're going to live together the rest of your life if you marry, so you figure the other person had better find out now what you're really like. Pretending most of the time creates too much tension and wears out a person.

f. You think chiefly of the satisfaction the other person can bring you.

g. Just a few things attract you to this person: maybe looks, maybe his "way with people," or maybe his personality.

h. Your parents think you need to wait longer before you let this relationship get serious. If you press them, they might tell you they doubt this is the one for you.

f. You think about how you can make the other person happy.

g. Many things attract you, besides looks. You share many common interests. You have the same values and the same life goals. You like to do things together. You enjoy spending time just talking with each other.

h. Your parents like your friend. They encourage you to get to know each other better. They suggest you invite your friend to share family times with you.

3. *What should you do when you see your boyfriend with another girl? Or your girlfriend with another boy?*

Let's turn that question around. A terrific guy you've been admiring finally asks you for a date. You have a wonderful evening. Before he takes you home, you stop for ice cream. Who should be there but the boy you've been dating rather steady lately. He sees you. The next time the two of you are together, how do you want him to treat you? Will your answer to this be the answer also to the question you asked?

4. *How should you handle the situation when your friend has a drug or alcohol problem?*

First, stop dating him. Second, see if you can convince your friend to get help. If you don't succeed, find other friends.

5. *How do you deal with this situation? You really liked someone once but lost interest. Now this person starts causing problems for you.*

The best solution is to do everything you can to stay out of sight of and avoid this person until he cools off and gets interested in someone else. If you can't avoid the person, make no comments at all in reply to his snide remarks. Let them wash over you like water. Most people will give up eventually if they are not successful in getting a response.

6. *How do you explain to someone that you don't want to see him anymore?*

You can say, "At our age we should get to know many people. We had a good time together, but now I'd rather get to know some others better. Maybe you also want to do this. At any rate, I do."

7. *How can you overcome shyness so you can talk to someone you like?*

You'll maybe find that once you plunge in and start talking, it will be so easy you'll wonder why you ever worried about it. Try working together on a project at school or church. Then you'll have a natural occasion to talk to each other. Sometimes it's easier to talk to each other over the phone. Or you can write a note asking if you can eat lunch together the next day.[1]

8. *How can you keep a relationship going when you live far apart?*

Not easy! There is the phone, of course, but someone has to pay those phone bills. Writing letters is better. In fact, you can get to know a person quite well through letter writing. If you are able to keep a relationship alive through letters and phone calls (letters mostly), you probably will want to see each other after a year. Maybe you could invite your friend to spend a week's vacation with your family at your home. Or the two of you could spend a week at the same camp.

9. *Why do kids today feel that sex is so important in their lives?*

Probably because most of them are influenced greatly by TV, movies, stories, pictures and ads. They are bombarded daily by sexual appeals that always make sex look glamorous, as if it were the answer to all problems. Add to this that in the teen years one becomes acutely aware of his own sexuality and his own sexual drive. That's pressure!

10. *How should you handle the situation when you and your best friend have liked the same guy, but he starts liking your friend—so your friend rubs it in your face about his liking her.*

That really hurts, doesn't it? It's like having a double-edged sword plunged into you and both edges of the sword ripping you apart.

Ask yourself this: Is a girl who rubs it into you worthy of being your best friend? She really is revealing a new side of her character by doing so, isn't she? Maybe you need to look for a new friend and let her go her way. In time she may see she has been wrong and come back to you and apologize. In the meantime, why not find someone else to be with?

---

[1]If shyness is a *big* problem for you, you might find it helpful to read *Why Am I Shy? Turning Shyness to Confidence* by Norman B. Rohrer and S. Philip Sutherland (Minneapolis: Augsburg Publishing House, 1978).

11. *What do you do when you think someone much older likes you?*

Go slowly. Go very slowly. When you get older, when you are in your mid-twenties or later, you can handle this situation better. For now, cool it. Why? Because older guys usually are more experienced, and if their motives aren't right, they can really lead you astray. It's flattering to have an older boyfriend, and therefore you might not be as wise or careful as you should. If the young man really likes you, he'll wait for you to get a little older.

12. *Why do kids make fun of you for liking someone of a different color?*

Probably they do that because either they feel very superior to someone of a different color or they feel uneasy about him, so this is their way of covering up their true feelings. Marriages between persons of mixed color do take place. Some are very happy marriages. Some are very sad. The problem doesn't come because of color (though in some communities that too is still a problem) but because of cultural patterns, habits, customs and value systems. The word in relationships of this nature is *Go slowly*, very slowly. Be sure you know each other very well. Be sure you can give in to each other. Be sure you can feel comfortable with the other person's family. Cross-cultural marriages can be enriching, but they are a big challenge. Not many can handle such a challenge successfully.

13. *I've been dating a boy who is of a different religion from ours. My parents are on to me about it. They say that I should date only kids who go to a Christian church. Why is that so important?*

Chances are, at your age, you aren't going to become serious about any boy you date. You undoubtedly will have a dozen or more boyfriends before you really settle on one. Nonetheless, you are establishing habits. Later on, whom you date will be very important. The more things people can have in common, the greater their chances are for a happy marriage. Religion, especially a Christian faith, can be one of the strongest bonding forces between two people, or in a family. Religion can also be very divisive. This is why your parents are concerned.

The Apostle Paul advised his Christian friends, "Do not be mismated with unbelievers." He then asked, "For what partnership have righteousness and iniquity?" (2 Cor. 6:14, RSV).

14. *A classmate at school is pregnant. She wants to keep the baby. She's starting to show now, and some of the kids at school are calling out, "Wow! Look at that bubble!" and "Here comes the elephant again," and all kinds of mean things. Others stand in a little cluster and talk and laugh and look at her. One of the kids from church says, "Well! Serves her right! She shouldn't have let it happen!" What is the best way to treat a girl like this? I'd like to be her friend.*

I'm glad you'd like to be her friend.

When our daughters were in high school, one of them came to me one day and said, "There's going to be a baby shower for Maureen [not her real name]," she said.

Maureen was our daughter's age. She wasn't married, and she didn't intend to get married. I sniffed and said in that horrible, smug tone that parents sometimes get, "Well! Do those who are giving the shower think that having a baby if you're not married is an occasion to celebrate?"

My daughter gave me a long look. Then she straightened up and said, "Mother, do you think the attitude you have is helping Maureen? She isn't happy either that it happened, and she wishes it hadn't, but she's determined to make the best of it. I'm going to her shower, and I'm going to buy her the nicest gift I can afford."

Do you know what I did? I went out and bought Maureen a gift too.

15. *If a girl gets pregnant, does that mean she has to get married?*

Years ago people thought if a girl became pregnant, she must marry, and she would sin even more if she didn't. Many girls did get married and spent the rest of their lives regretting it.

We all make mistakes, and in rebellion against God we all have sinned. But to marry someone whom we don't really love, and even to marry when we are very young is just making one mistake after another. Girls and fellows who get into this situation should discuss the future with their parents and their pastors, and make decisions, slowly, prayerfully and carefully.[2]

---

[2]An excellent resource for a teen-aged girl who finds herself pregnant is *Should I Keep My Baby?* by Martha Zimmerman (Minneapolis: Bethany House Publishers, 1983).

What Would You Say?

Debbie is 14 years old. She thinks she is in love with Rick, 17, who has been dating her for two months. They are together during all their free time. Debbie says she can't think of anything besides Rick. Her parents, however, tell her she is only infatuated with Rick, that she doesn't really love him.

So Debbie asks you, "How can I know whether or not I'm in love?"

How would you answer her? What questions could you ask her? After you've written down your questions, turn to the next page and read some of the questions we suggest.

Questions to ask Debbie

Here are some questions you should ask Debbie:
1. What do you like about Rick?
2. When did you begin to like Rick?
3. Why did you become interested in him?
4. How long have you really liked each other?
5. How has your romance affected your schoolwork? Your life at home? Your disposition?
6. Do your parents like Rick? Explain.
7. What have Rick and you done together?
8. If you couldn't see Rick for six months, what would you do? Would you seek out other friends?
9. Do Rick and you sometimes disagree and fight? About what? How do you make up?
10. How do you feel when you see Rick talking to and paying attention to another girl? How do you act?
11. If Rick asked you to do something which you don't like, would you still do it to please him?

What does Debbie like about Rick? The way he looks? The way he dresses? The car he drives? People's looks change as they grow older. They might not be able to continue to dress as nicely once they have to earn their own money. Besides, these are just outward things. People are more than just faces and bodies and legs. People are personalities. Pretty girls or handsome boys may not be beautiful people. Beautiful people may not be good-looking or sharp dressers. Real beauty comes from the *inside*. But with all the emphasis placed on figures and good looks, it's hard to remember this.

Debbie says she has known Rick only two months. Getting to know someone, however, takes a long, long time. A person may act wonderfully on a date (who doesn't?) but be a witch or a monster at home. How does this friend treat his parents and sisters and brothers? How does he act when asked to do chores? When he gets sick? When his plans don't work out? When he loses a game? When somebody criticizes him? It takes time to see a person in each of these situations. Can you still love and respect that person when he or she is grumpy, depressed, irritable, unkind and hard to get along with? It is important to ask these questions, because life lasts a long, long time, and after you are married you can be sure you will find yourselves in all these, and even more difficult situations.

True love makes us better people all the way around. We become more thoughtful and considerate of everybody, and willing to help. True love doesn't make us neglectful of others.

An old Korean proverb says that parents see farther because they have lived longer. Parents love their kids more than anybody else, and good parents want only the best for their children. Because of that we don't have to be afraid of asking our parents what they think of our friends, and it isn't a bad idea at all to listen to what they have to say either.

What is Debbie's motive? Is she asking, "What can I get out of this?" or is she thinking, "What can I do to make Rick a better person?" True love is unselfish. Infatuation is selfish, on the lookout only for one's self. Many young people have ten or twelve cases of puppy love or infatuation before they really begin to love. So maybe you should say to Debbie, "Cool it."

Is Romantic Love the Only Answer to Loneliness?

Joanna is 18 years old. She is attractive, intelligent and a Christian. But Joanna feels very sad because she has never had a date. She feels she must not be desirable or attractive, and therefore she isn't worthwhile. She has periods of great loneliness. She wishes and wishes she could have a boyfriend. This has become so important to her that she spends much time brooding over it.

Discussion

1. Why do you think Joanna feels she is not worthwhile?
2. Would having a boyfriend necessarily take care of her loneliness?
3. Are kids who date sometimes lonely? Why?
4. Are married people sometimes lonely? Why?
5. If romantic, sexual love is only one expression of God's love, how else may we love others and be loved?
6. What would help Joanna?

Teen-agers Define Love

How would you define love? Write a paragraph about it below. Then read what other teen-agers wrote.

Love is:

"Love means seeing faults in a person but accepting them."

"Love means you want to do things for the other person. You try to make the other person happy."

"Love is made up of respect, of self-esteem, of happiness and of satisfaction in life."

"Love is a relationship of being able to get along well with another person and being able to endure everything that happens because that person is with you."

"Love includes affection, friendliness, recognition, approval, acceptance and esteem."

"Love is consideration for the other person and what both would like to accomplish. It is give and take. It is being patient continually and abounding in thoughtfulness."

"Love is belonging. Love is an attraction to another's ideas, thoughts and standards."

"Love is willingness to make sacrifices and allowances for another's faults or failures."

"Love means being able to share not only one's happy experiences but also one's disappointments, griefs and one's innermost feelings with the assurance that these feelings will be respected and what is told will be kept in confidence."

"Love is a relationship which grows and takes time to grow."

"Love is learning to cooperate and adjust."

"Love means feeling the pain and happiness of the other person."

"Love is caring enough to be able to spend your entire life with that person."

"Love means being able to forgive."

"You know you're in love when you get all dressed up to meet her Aunt Gladys from Pittsburgh."[3]

One girl thought the Apostle Paul gave the best description of love.

> Love is very patient and kind, never jealous or envious, never boastful or proud, never haughty or selfish or rude. Love does not demand its own way. It is not irritable or touchy. It does not hold grudges and will hardly even notice when others do it wrong. It is never glad about injustice, but rejoices whenever truth wins out. If you love someone, you will be loyal to him no matter what the cost. You will always believe in him, always expect the best of him, and always stand your ground in defending him. (1 Cor. 13:4–7, TLB)

After reading this, are you better able to understand the difference between infatuation and love?

---

[3]Answers are excerpted from *Ideas and Learning Activities for Family Life and Sex Education* by Mark Perrin and Thomas E. Smith (Dubuque, Iowa: Wm. B. Brown Co., Publishers). Used by permission.

7 ❖ WHY WAIT UNTIL MARRIAGE TO HAVE SEX?

1. *Why is premarital sex wrong?*

Why did you ask that question the way you did? It makes me think you already believe it is. But let me give you my answer.

I could mention many things. I could talk about the high risk of contracting a disease that could damage you for life. Diseases caught through sexual intercourse are common among teen-agers. If you don't know a person very well, you can't be sure he or she is not a carrier.

I could talk about your losing the joy of telling your husband or wife—when you finally are ready to be married—that you have waited to be his or hers alone. That's special.

If you are thinking of premarital sex with someone you plan to marry, I could mention the risk you run of finding your relationship doesn't last until your wedding day. And then comes the disappointment that your virginity is gone. Statistics show that those who engage in premarital sex do not have as great a chance at a truly happy marriage as those who don't.

I could mention the real possibility of pregnancy.

I could remind you that if word gets around that you are doing this, you could lose the chance of a really great relationship with someone who wants a girl or fellow who believes in being sexually pure.

I could ask you how your parents would feel if you did this. What would this do to your relationship with them?

I could ask if you can be sure of not feeling guilty afterward, and if you do, what will you do with that guilt?

I could remind you that memories have a way of sticking with us and haunting us. Will these actions be good memories for you five or ten years from now?

There's an awful lot to think about, isn't there? And some of these things are heavy considerations. Still there's a remote possibility that you could come up with a satisfactory (at least to your way of thinking) answer to all these questions. So where does that leave us?

What does God say?

In the Bible, sexual intercourse outside the marriage union is called "fornication." From Genesis right through Revelation an awful lot is said about fornication, either directly or through stories.[1] In Old Testament times it was regarded as being so serious that a person could be put to death for it! The least punishment was for a boy to marry the girl and never, never divorce her (Deut. 22:13–29). What would happen if we enforced that today?

In Romans 1:29 Paul lists fornication along with murder and ruthlessness. In Galatians 5:19–21 he lists it along with jealousy, drunkenness, carousing and other sins. As we read the Bible we cannot miss the message that God forbids sexual intercourse outside of marriage. He does this, not because He's an old ogre who wants to make things difficult and unpleasant for us. He does this because He loves us and wants to protect us. He knows far better than we do the heartache and sorrow that can come from broken relationships, disease, unwanted children and abused, neglected children. God isn't against sex. Sex is one of His gracious gifts to us. But He doesn't want us to use the gift selfishly and disregard His law.

Maybe we need to go a step further and ask yet another question. God has commanded us to live pure lives. Read Galatians 5:16–24; 1 Corinthians 6:9–10; Romans 12:1; 1 Peter 1:15. If we do not obey God's commands, what does this say about our relationship to God? Jesus said we prove we love Him if we _____. (Look up His words in John 14:15.)

The Apostle John underscored this same point: "And by this we may be sure that we know him, if we keep his commandments. He who says 'I know him' but disobeys his commandments is a liar" (1 John 2:3, RSV). Later he writes, "For this is the love of God, that we keep his commandments" (1 John 5:3, RSV).

These verses show how serious it is if we willfully and con-

---

[1] Genesis includes no direct statement about fornication, but it shows the trouble caused by sex outside of marriage (Gen. 16, 21, 38).

sciously disobey and continue to disobey God's commands, for when we do this we prove we do not know Him and do not love Him. So then, committing the sin of fornication is sin, not only against ourselves and others, but against God. It is telling God that we don't love Him, and we don't want to be His.

2. *My older sister is engaged. She and I talk a lot. She says I shouldn't even think of having sex because I'm just a kid (I'm 14), and I'm not ready for marriage. But she says it's all right for her to have sex because she's engaged. Is she right?*

No. Being engaged isn't the same as being married. When you get engaged you tell your friends and family and the public that you *intend* to marry. But the time of engagement is a waiting time, a testing time. Sometimes engaged couples decide they don't want to live a lifetime together. Then they break their engagement. If they had sex during the time they were engaged but later decided not to get married, can it be anything other than fornication?

E. M. Blaiklock, a noted biblical scholar, insists that the New Testament writers did not consider any sexual act outside the formal covenant of marriage as acceptable, that they included under fornication "all sex experiences outside the one legitimate occasion—marriage." He goes on to say: "There is not a phrase or word in the New Testament which in any way condones extra-marital sex. . . . The whole force of the New Testament is behind chastity and the sanctity of marriage."[2] He points out that, in 1 Corinthians 7:9, 36, Paul told the Corinthian Christians that if the sex desire during courtship became too strong, they should marry so they would not fall into the sin of fornication. To insist on intercourse before marriage, therefore, is to place one's own will and pleasure before obedience to God.

Young people should also learn not to expect too much from sex. It can be great, but it also can be ordinary, and sometimes even disappointing. It often takes time to develop a sex life that is satisfying and pleasurable to both the husband and wife. But in marriage the couple can relax and take the necessary time. They understand that their decision to love each other above all others is the most important ingredient of their relation-

[2]Matt. 5:32; 15:19; 19:9; Mark 7:21; Acts 15:20, 29; 21:25; Rom. 1:29; 1 Cor. 5:1, 9, 10; 6:9, 13, 18; 7:2; 10:8; 2 Cor. 12:21; Gal. 5:19; Eph. 5:3; Col. 3:5; 1 Thess. 4:3; Heb. 13:4; Jude 7; Rev. 2:14, 20; 9:20, 21.

ship. Having made this decision, they don't need to fear that the spouse will walk out just because there are some difficulties to work through. It's much easier for an engaged couple to call it quits than for a married couple. So having intercourse before marriage actually can work against a permanent, joy-filled relationship.

Often, too, when engaged couples begin to have sex, this consumes all their attention, and they don't spend time getting to know each other better in preparation for marriage. It can't be said too often that marriage carries more meaning than just the physical union of two people.

But the most important thing to remember is that, according to God's Word, sex is reserved for the married couple.

3. *But how can persons know they will be happy together sexually if they don't try and also practice?*

There are some skills that require practice, but sex is different from playing tennis or the piano. You don't have to have sex with three, four or a dozen people in order to "become good at it." In fact, the more people you have sex with the less your chances become of ever having a permanent, satisfying sex life.

In the first place, each person is different. Just because you've been "good at sex" with one person is no guarantee you're going to be "good at it" with everybody else.

In the second place, we need to understand that many factors contribute to whether or not sex between two people will be a good experience. It is important that the two share in the same values. It helps if they have had comparable educational training and hold similar intellectual understandings. They need to have some interests in common, whether they be in music, writing, reading, sports, traveling, photography, entertaining, or whatever. Having all interests in common is not necessary. In fact, to have one or two differing interests can add spice and variety to their life together. But the couple needs to have enough in common so they can spend time together pleasurably.

No, enjoyable sex with a person does not guarantee a happy married life. But compatability in many areas, that is, enjoying the same things and having the same interests, values and goals, leads to a satisfying sexual life. So don't experiment with sex, believing that this will show you whether or not marriage to that person would be good. Premarital sex is a wretched test.

If you have a good, loving relationship with another, if you share much in common, if you are frank and honest with each other, and if you have no severe sexual problems (emotional or physical), your chance of having a satisfying sexual life together is excellent. Practice or experimenting is not necessary. Don't do it.

4. *If premarital sex is so wrong, why are so many doing it?*

For many reasons. One of the chief reasons, especially for young people, is that it seems "everybody is doing it," and if you don't, you'll be the weird one. Of course, everyone is not doing it. It just seems that way. Actually more are not doing it than are. And it still remains true (according to surveys) that the majority of people say they want to marry someone who hasn't had sex with others.

Second, kids think premarital sex is commonly accepted as permissible. Movies, ads, TV all tell us this. Without question we really are deeply affected by what we see and hear over and over. After something has been repeated often enough we'll begin to believe it. The sad part is that the media often doesn't tell us the truth. People still respect most highly those who live morally pure lives.

Third, it's easier to prevent pregnancies now than it used to be, so kids feel safer. And if one gets pregnant, kids think the girl always can get an abortion. They don't realize the pain and anguish that accompany abortion. (More on this in chapter 9.)

Fourth, some kids have such a gloomy outlook on life that they think the world might not hang together much longer, so they're going to have "fun" while they can. This really isn't a new excuse. In every age some have given this as a reason for living as they want to.

Fifth, It's easier now to find a place to have sex because in so many homes both parents work and kids come home from school to an empty house. More kids own cars too. And if you're in college, dorms are shared by both men and women, making access to rooms easy.

Sixth, kids think their parents won't get too mad if they find out because so many other parents' kids have behaved in this way. It seems no one is too terribly embarrassed anymore. It isn't hidden. People talk about it. All that some Christian parents say is, "Pray for us." Some seem resigned to it. What kids don't realize is that behind this "brave" front of parents there is a lot of hurt and disappointment. I haven't met any parents yet who have felt good that their kids have had sex outside of marriage.

Seventh, some churches have become very permissive in their teachings on extramarital sex. As one young girl said, "We hear on every hand that it is all right. We need to hear just as many voices saying it is not all right, and we don't hear those voices— not even in church."

5. *Sex is just exercise, so what's wrong with it?*

Sorry, sex isn't just exercise. Sex involves the most intimate contact you can have with another person. Sex carries the possibility of bringing into being another life. No other exercise does that.

Exercise is meant to benefit us physically. Sex, rightly used, can relieve tension. But sex misused causes many physical problems as well as diseases.

6. *Sex is the one good thing in my life. If I didn't have it, I would be alone and lonely. I wouldn't have any social life and all the kids would think I'm strange.*

My heart aches for you. You need to find friends and develop some other interests and skills. What do you enjoy doing? Sports? Music? Swimming? Art? Is there a church near you which has a youth program? If you can find a group of young people who have fun playing together, helping others and worshiping together, your interest in sex will become much less important. It will assume its rightful place in your life.

Friendship with other kids will ease some of the loneliness you feel. Even more, coming to know the Lord Jesus as your Friend, Savior and Helper will take care of the loneliness. Many years ago a wise man wrote that God has created us for Himself and our hearts are restless until they find rest in God. That statement is still true today. Find a church home.

7. *My friend Nancy was in love with a guy named Rick. Rick talked her into having sex with him one night. But the next time they dated Rick started to make fun of her and laugh at her, and finally they quarreled so much they had to cut their date short. Nancy says it's been like that every time they get together now. What's happened? Nancy says before they had sex Rick was really nice to her, and she was sure he loved her.*

Girls usually don't enter into a sexual relationship unless

they feel an emotional or romantic attachment to the boy. Boys, on the other hand, can be casual and have sex with a girl for whom they feel no strong romantic pull. However, after they have had sex with a girl they often feel guilty. They feel they seduced the girl. To cover up their guilt they begin to belittle the girl and quarrel. If the girl then breaks off the relationship, they feel cleared of guilt.

Girls need to be aware that, generally speaking, they become emotionally involved more quickly than fellows. Because of this they misinterpret boys' actions and words, reading more into them than they should, and often wind up being hurt. Boys who are aware of this female tendency often draw back when they notice it happening; thus the girl deprives herself of what maybe could become a meaningful relationship because the boy, not wanting to hurt the girl, does not feel free to develop the friendship further.

Peer Pressure

Why do so many teen-agers get involved in sexual relations even when they really don't want to or when they really don't enjoy it?

Dr. James Dobson, in *Preparing for Adolescence*, states one of the reasons is peer pressure. If everybody else in a group is doing something, you don't want to be the single, lone oddball who doesn't do it, do you?

He relates an experiment some doctors conducted to examine the influence of "but everybody's doing it." The doctors invited ten teen-agers to participate in a test that supposedly would test their visual perception. The doctors said they would show a number of cards, each with a straight line drawn on it. The students were to indicate which card had the longer line. All the students were seated almost equally close to the instructor. But previous to their entering the room, nine of the students had been instructed to raise their hand when the card with the *shorter* line was held up.

The test began. The instructor picked out two cards. The first one had the shorter line. Nine of the students promptly indicated it was the card with the longer line. The tenth student looked puzzled, but when all nine persisted with their hands up and stared at him, he too finally raised his hand. Again and again in the course of the test the same thing happened, with the tenth student, looking perplexed, but hesitantly voting with the others.

They took a break. Then one of the nine was instructed to object and insist the other line was the longer. When this happened, the tenth student quickly sided with the student who was pointing out the error.

The test was conducted with a number of teen-agers. Only five out of every 20 students tested had the courage to vote alone against the crowd.

The test showed the immense influence others have on us. When we are in a group, we don't want to be different.

But the test also showed the effect that just *one* person disagreeing can have on a group. Then others dare to stand up for what they really believe.

Discussion

1. Do you believe that peer pressure of this kind is a major reason why teens engage is sex? Or do you disagree? Explain.
2. Discuss ways in which peer pressure has affected you.
3. How could giving in to peer pressure get you into trouble? Explain.
4. How could giving in to peer pressure affect your whole life?
5. When we give in to peer pressure, what does it show that we need to develop in our lives?
6. Not only teen-agers have trouble with peer pressure. Adults do too. Sometimes they resist the pressure and stand up for what they believe is right. Sometimes they give in and are sorry later, or else they suffer because they don't like themselves for not sticking up for what they believe. Read Daniel 1. How did Daniel and his friends feel the pressure being put on them? What was the outcome of their resistance to the pressure?
7. Now read Daniel 6. What new pressure was on Daniel? Why, do you think, did the presidents and governors decide to put the pressure on Daniel? What did the presidents and governors know would give Daniel courage to disobey even the king's edict? (see verse 5). This time, what happened to Daniel when he refused to follow the crowd? Ultimately, how did God defend Daniel?
8. Read Matthew 26:69–75. Why do you think Peter did what

he did? What was the result of his action?

9. What does God's Word have to say to *us*? Read Romans 12:2. "Don't copy the behavior and customs of this world, but be a new and different person with a fresh newness in all you do and think. Then you will learn from your own experience how his ways will really satisfy you" (TLB).

10. What does the Bible say might be the consequence of our not going along with the crowd? (Read 1 John 3:13.) If this happens, what should we remember? (Read John 15:18–21.)

What Would You Do?

(Answers on next page)

It's a good idea to imagine certain scenes and situations and think what choices you would have in that situation. Then if you ever find yourself in that situation, you already will have thought it through and will know how to act. You won't be carried away by the emotions of the moment and later regret your action. Remember always that you can choose and decide what you want to do.

Consider the following situation.

Sandra and Karl are in Karl's car. It's their first date. Sandra knows that Karl had sexual relations with his other girlfriends, and she is worried. She thinks Karl is headed for a park and will want to make love. Sandra doesn't want to make love. What can Sandra say or do?

(If you wish, you may turn to the next page for some alternatives we suggest that Sandra could consider.)

What Would You Say?

(Answers on next page)

Denise and Joel have been going steady for several months. Denise thinks that she loves Joel. She wants to please him. Above all, she doesn't want to lose him. Lately Joel has been becoming more and more intimate. Finally he asks her for sex. She stalls.

He says, "If you love me, then prove it by having sex with me."

How can Denise answer Joel?

Our Answers to What Would You Do?

1. Sandra can suggest they go somewhere else, such as a pizza parlor or ice cream place.
2. She can tell Karl she has to be and wants to be home in ten minutes.
3. She can ask Karl outright where they are going and what he wants to do. She can then tell him plainly she doesn't want to go. She can also say, "You might as well know right from the beginning that I don't believe in heavy petting or going all the way. I just want to be friends and have a good time. Getting involved in sex isn't my idea of having a good time."

Question to discuss: Why can deciding there will be no sexual relationship outside of marriage bring a sense of relief to a couple when they are dating?

Our Answers to What Would You Say?

1. Denise can say, "Now I know you don't really love me or you wouldn't ask me for this."
2. She can say, "Learn to know me and discover my best qualities. Let me learn to know you. If you insist on rushing, I'll be forced to believe there isn't much worthy in you. I want to wait for sex until I am married."

Question to discuss: What if, after Denise gives these or similar answers, the relationship breaks up? How can Denise handle this?

Agree or Disagree?

Why does a boy try to have sex with a girl he doesn't know very well and whom he doesn't really love? What answers would you give to that question?

Walter Trobisch, in his book *I Married You*, gives three of his answers:

1. He is afraid that unless he has sex he will become sick or neurotic or both.
2. He thinks he has to learn by doing.
3. He wants to brag about his conquest.

Do you agree or disagree with him? Discuss his answers. If you agree or disagree, tell why you do.

Agree or Disagree?

Why would a girl give herself to a boy whom she hardly knows and for whom she does not care deeply? What answers would you give to that question? Here are some answers that have been suggested:

1. She thinks having intercourse is proof she is worldly-wise and attractive.

2. She looks upon intercourse as "payment" for the date.

3. Everybody does it. If she doesn't, others will think she is weird and abnormal.

4. She is afraid the boy will drop her if she doesn't consent.

5. She says it's a natural thing to do if you care for each other at all.

6. She says it is impossible to have a meaningful relationship without sex.

7. She wants to bind the boy to her.

8. Consciously or unconsciously she wants a baby.

Do you agree or disagree? Discuss these answers. If you agree or disagree, tell why you do.

True or False

(Answers on next page)

1. _____ Romantic love is *the* answer to feeling alone, rejected and worthless.

2. _____ Developing new skills, whether they be in physical sports or in crafts, mechanics, music, art, etc., helps put sex in the proper perspective.

3. _____ When people use sex to control another, it is usually because they feel insecure.

4. _____ To view sexual organs of the opposite sex is harmless if you are not married.

5. _____ Talking about sex is dirty.

6. _____ Put-downs destroy communication.

7. _____ Talking about sex will lead to experimenting with sex.

Answers to True or False

1. *False.* Romantic love is only one expression of love. Becoming involved with a group in which we are accepted, loved and cherished also meets our feelings of loneliness.

2. *True.* Developing a number of new skills helps put sex in its proper perspective. Sex is only one expression of the creative powers God has given us. It is only one way to develop and nourish a feeling of closeness and unity with another. It is a wonderful gift, but it is only one gift.

3. *True.* A secure person respects others and will not use them. A secure person desires the best for the other person. A marriage runs into trouble when a spouse uses sex to manipulate, by withholding sex as punishment, or giving sex as a reward.

4. *False.* To view sexual organs makes us vulnerable and open to temptation because it can stimulate our desires and break down our resistance.

5. *False.* Talking about sex can be dirty, but it need not be. God created sex and sexuality, so they are good. Understanding sexuality teaches us to marvel at our God-given creative powers and the amazing way God has created our bodies.

6. *True.* Put-downs always destroy communication. Building positive feelings and affirming another encourages communication.

7. *False.* Those who want to experiment with sex will do so regardless of what is said and done. On the other hand, accurate information about sexual matters can help a person make wise decisions and avoid unnecessary experimentation.

Bible Study

(Answers on next page)

Carefully read 1 Corinthians 6:12–20 in two or three versions that are easy to understand. Then answer the following questions.

1. Some Corinthian Christians said having sex outside of marriage was as natural as eating and drinking. What did Paul say in answer to this?
2. What does Paul say about our bodies? As Christians, to whom are we joined? To whom do our bodies belong?

3. How does Paul describe the Christian's body?
4. How much did Christ pay to purchase us?

Answers to Bible Study

1. Paul says very clearly that the body was not meant to be used for immorality, that is, it wasn't meant to be used for sexually impure acts (v. 13).

2. Paul says that our bodies belong to Christ, that our bodies are precious and that even after death God will raise them up (vv. 14, 15).

3. Paul says that we are one with Christ, and that if we act immorally, if we sin sexually, we sin against our own bodies. He says we are to flee immorality. He describes our bodies as being temples in which the Holy Spirit dwells, the Holy Spirit whom God has sent to us. Therefore we are not our own. We belong to God (vv. 17–19).

4. Jesus gave the dearest that He had to purchase us so we could belong to God. He gave His own life. How we treat our bodies and how we use our bodies will reflect how much we love Jesus and how grateful we are to Him for all that He has done for us (v. 20).

Discussion

1. How can romantic love become either a beautiful expression of God's love or a perversion?
2. How might people use sex to control others?
3. Are kids abnormal if they don't want to have sex until they are married?
4. How does language color what we say?
5. When is touch an expression of love? of lust?
6. With whom are you comfortable discussing sex? Why are you uncomfortable talking with some people about sex? What are you afraid some people will say or do?
7. What don't you understand about love and sex but wish you had more information?
8. What have the TV shows you watched this last week told you about sex?
9. In one episode on the TV show *M*A*S*H*, Hawkeye Pierce was seducing an army nurse. As they murmured sweet nothings to each other she happened to make a disparaging re-

mark about Koreans. Hawkeye, in disgust, left the tent. What was the double message given to the viewer? What TV shows have you seen lately that have given similar messages? How can this affect us?

Checklist for Self-esteem

Surveys and interviews have shown that people who have a healthy self-esteem are not as interested in extramarital sex as those who do not think highly of themselves. God wants us to see ourselves as He sees us. We are His magnificent creation. And even though we have sinned, we can be forgiven in Christ and deeply loved by God as His children. Because of this we should be able to stand tall—humbly.

How do you regard yourself? On the following list, check if you received from someone (preferably your parents) during the last couple days . . .

1. a word of praise.
2. a hug.
3. the words, "I love you."
4. help with your homework.
5. a listening ear so you could talk about what had happened during the day or what was troubling you or making you happy.

Now on the list below, check if during the last couple of days in your relationship with your parents you . . .

1. praised them.
2. hugged or kissed them.
3. told them you loved them.
4. asked them how their day was.
5. helped with house or yard work.

Discuss your findings with your parents. Talk and pray. Then let your mother and dad tell about something you have done or said that has meant a lot to them or made them proud of you. Afterward you do the same for them.

Agree or Disagree

(Answers on next page)

Discuss the following statements and tell why you agree or disagree.

1. Women's sexual needs are as great as men's.

2. The percentage of people having sex outside of marriages is much greater now than it was 50 years ago.

3. Sex was not emphasized in Bible times. People were not tempted as much as they are today.

4. Remaining sexually pure is more difficult today than years ago.

Answers to Agree or Disagree

1. *Women's sexual needs are as great as men's.*

This is true, though it is commonly said that men have greater needs than women so it is all right for men to have sexual affairs outside of marriage while it is wrong for women to do so. Not true! Women long for intimate relationships, for assurance of being loved and for close body contact with a man as much as men do.

2. *The percentage of people having sex outside of marriages is much greater now than it was 50 years ago.*

During the 19th century about one-fourth of all the brides had experienced sexual relations before they were married. During the 1920s this figure jumped to 50%. It has remained pretty close to this until the present time, although some sociologists think it may take a 10% jump during this decade.

3. *Sex was not emphasized in Bible times. People were not tempted as they are today.*

People always have been tempted by illicit sex. The age we live in is not exceptional. In the Bible, having sex before marriage is referred to as "fornication." The word appears at least 60 times in the Bible. (Footnote 2 in this chapter lists only some of the New Testament references to premarital and extramarital sex.) That should tell us something about how common that sin was in those days and how strongly God spoke against it.

In many of the religions where Jehovah God was not worshiped, sex was worshiped. Followers carved images of sexual organs. Some of the Greek deities were gods and goddesses who encouraged sexual relations of every kind outside of marriage. It is said that there were so many prostitutes in Ephesus (location of the temple of Diana) during New Testament times, and they made so much money from their business, that when the city had to borrow money they borrowed from the prostitutes.

4. *Remaining sexually pure is more difficult today than years ago.*

The people of Israel grew up among a people who thought nothing of having sexual relations outside of marriage. Yet God commanded His people to remain morally pure (Ex. 20:14; Lev. 20:10; Deut. 22:13–24). His command to us today is the same. Can we legitimately say that it is any harder? That our times are worse or that it is more difficult for us to remain pure? Every age has been characterized with temptations to sin. There never has been a time when living pure lives has not been difficult. And it continues to be difficult. Even if we attend Christian schools there will always be some people who will tempt us to do wrong. And the movies and TV we see, and the stories we read, and the talk that we hear constantly will tempt us to do wrong. But God has promised to make us strong and to provide for us, when the temptation comes, a way of escape. To say that it is harder for us today to remain sexually pure is just a lazy excuse, a looking for a way out of being obedient to God.

Before You Go into a House Where Nobody's Home or Get in the Backseat of a Car—THINK

Jeffrey and Jennifer are twins. They always have been close to each other, and now, even in their adolescent years, they continue to talk about things together.

Both of them are sure they don't want to get mixed up with sex before they are married. One day they sat down and made out a long list of everything they could think of that would help them keep their resolve. Each of them had experienced a couple of crushes and heartbreaks, so they knew a little about how overpowering emotions can become. Neither of them, however, had a crush on anyone at this time, so it was easier for them to think about the subject objectively.

Before you read their list, however, take ten minutes to make out your own list. What can you do that will help you say no when you are tempted to "go all the way"? Ask your parents to make out a list of suggestions too. Compare the lists and discuss them.

Now turn to Jeffrey and Jennifer's list. Evaluate their guidelines as "very important," "good idea" or "not necessary." Afterward give reasons for your evaluations.

To protect my sexual purity . . .	Very important	Good idea	Not necessary
I will not get into a backseat of a parked car with my friend.	☐	☐	☐

I will not allow myself to be led to thick shrubbery or lie on the ground in a secluded area. ☐ ☐ ☐

I will not be in my friend's bedroom at any time without the door being wide open. ☐ ☐ ☐

I will not go inside any house with my friend if the parents are not home. ☐ ☐ ☐

I will not explore under a girl's clothing (Jeffrey's resolve). ☐ ☐ ☐

I will not allow a boy to explore under my clothing (Jennifer's resolve). ☐ ☐ ☐

I will never undress in front of my friend or be undressed with my friend. ☐ ☐ ☐

I will never allow myself to be tightly glued against the body of my friend for more than a few brief minutes. Even ten minutes is too long. I will break away often and maintain some distance. ☐ ☐ ☐

When our friendship begins to deepen, I will let my friend know early that I do not believe in heavy petting or sex before marriage. ☐ ☐ ☐

I will not travel with my friend on an automobile trip unless someone else accompanies us. ☐ ☐ ☐

I will not go to movies that arouse me sexually or look at pornographic pictures. ☐ ☐ ☐

I will work hard at having several friends and doing things with them. ☐ ☐ ☐

I will try to maintain good relationships with my parents and pray for openness to talk with them. ☐ ☐ ☐

If I can't establish this openness with my parents, I will try to find one or two adults, who are understanding and who cherish Christian values, in whom I can confide. ☐ ☐ ☐

I will look forward with joy to the day when I am ready to assume the responsibilities of marriage, when I can join my heart and life with another.

☐ ☐ ☐

I will constantly play this recorded message in my mind: "I am keeping myself for the one I shall marry one day."

☐ ☐ ☐

If my friends begin to have sex with their dates, I'll drop those friends and look for others.

☐ ☐ ☐

I shall try to maintain a quiet time of prayer and Bible reading every day.

☐ ☐ ☐

I shall continue to attend church regularly and find some area in the church where I can be active.

☐ ☐ ☐

I won't go away for weekend trips alone with my friend.

☐ ☐ ☐

I won't date guys who have a reputation for easy sex (Jennifer's resolve).

☐ ☐ ☐

I will keep telling myself: "You're not alone. Lots of other kids want to remain virgins."

☐ ☐ ☐

I will choose my friends carefully. I won't get too "thick" with anyone until I really know the person.

☐ ☐ ☐

Should I or Shouldn't I?

So you're wondering if you should or shouldn't. Should you get involved in heavy petting? How about that neat guy who wants you to sleep with him? Or the one who wants you to go steady with him? Should you be using contraceptives? Should I or shouldn't I? The questions churn around in your mind.

Here are some questions to ask yourself when faced with a situation that demands a decision. They're from the book *Be Good to Each Other* by Lowell and Carol Erdahl.[3] Don't rush

---

[3]Lowell and Carol Erdahl, *Be Good to Each Other* (New York: Harper and Row, Publishers, Inc., 1981). Used by permission.

through these questions. Pray before you answer. Think carefully about each one.

1. *The law test:* Is it (the contemplated action) in accordance with the Ten Commandments?

2. *The Golden Rule test:* Is it in accordance with the Golden Rule, "Do unto others as you would have them do unto you"?

3. *The test of Jesus' new commandment:* Is it in accord with Jesus' new commandment to "love one another as I have loved you"?

4. *The test of consequences:* Is it hurtful or helpful to myself and others?

5. *The test of publicity:* Is it something I'd be pleased to have everyone know about?

6. *The test of respect:* Is it something I'd like those whom I respect the most to know about?

7. *The test of universality:* Would the world be better or worse if everyone were to act in the way I'm thinking of acting?

8. *The test of projected retrospect:* Will I likely be pleased five/ten years from now to have done what I'm thinking of doing today?

9. *The test of Jesus' example:* Is it something Jesus would do?

10. *The test of self-love:* Does it express equal love of neighbor as of self? If I do this, will I be caring as much for others as I care for myself?

11. *The test of conscience:* Will I feel regret or gratitude after the deed is done or left undone?

Bible Study

(Answers on next page)

Prayerfully read 1 Thessalonians 4:1–18 in two or three versions that are easy to understand. Then answer the following questions.

1. What does Paul beg the Christians in Thessalonica to do?
2. What does Paul say the will of God is?
3. What does the word "holy" mean?
4. What does the word "fornication" mean?
5. What does Paul say about fornication (also translated unchastity, immorality, or sexual sin)?
6. How does Paul say the Christians are to remain sexually pure? How can they do it?
7. What is the difference between lust and love?
8. How will God deal with those who disobey?
9. God wants us to be sexually pure. When we aren't, against whom are we rebelling?
10. According to these verses, how are we to be different from those who do not know Christ?
11. "No man must do his brother wrong in this matter, or invade his rights" (v. 6, NEB). How can we harm others by how we act sexually?
12. What has God promised to give us to help us live pure lives?

Answers to Bible Study

1. Paul begs the Christians in Thessalonica to walk and behave in a way that will please God (v. 1). He says they have done this in the past and he tells them to continue. In fact, he says, they are to excel in their effort to please God—to go all out—to go for it! And they are to do this more and more.

2. Paul says that it is the will of God that they be people set apart for Him, people who do not have sex outside of marriage.

3. The word "holy" means to be set apart for God, to choose to be His, to choose to obey Him.

4. The word "fornication" is the word used in the Bible to describe sexual relations outside of marriage.

5. Paul says that fornication is giving way to lustful passion, to want something for oneself and to want it no matter what God says or no matter whether or not it brings harm to anyone else.

6. (Verse 8.) Paul says that God knows we are weak and so He has given us the Holy Spirit to live in us and empower us to do that which pleases Him. We can trust the Holy Spirit.

7. Lust means that I see someone whom I want to possess and enjoy for my own fulfillment, and I want to do it right away. Love means that I give priority to the happiness and the good of the other person, and I am willing to wait until the time is right for both of us.

8. Paul solemnly warns the Christians in Thessalonica that God is an avenger; that is, when we do wrong, things have a way of coming back to us and we suffer for what we have done.

9. In verse 8 Paul says that when we don't live lives that are sexually pure we are rejecting God, rebelling against God, turning up our nose at God. We are saying that we know better than He, that we don't care what He says, that we are going to do what we want to do. We are closing our ears to what God is saying to us. We are turning our backs on Him and saying we don't care that He loved us enough to die for us.

10. Paul says that those who do not know God give themselves over to lustful passions; that is, they carry on sexually in any way they wish. Paul says that Christians respect their bodies (v. 4) and they keep them pure for God; they honor God by doing so.

11. If we have sex with others outside of marriage, we can

rob them of their purity. If a boy gets a girl pregnant, he robs her of her freedom. She has to decide how she will care for the baby to whom she gives birth. Some give disease to others through their sexual acts, disease that causes blindness or sometimes even insanity. (More about that in chapter 10.) At the very least, boys and girls alike may feel guilty and unhappy, and even if they get married later on, memories will remain with them. So you see, we can harm others in many, many ways by how we behave sexually. I'm sure you can think of many more ways (e.g., broken relationships that result between parents and children because parents are disappointed).

12. God has commanded us to live morally pure lives, and He has given us His Holy Spirit to live in us and control us, to make it possible to obey Him.

Dear Abby on Proving Love by Consenting to Have Sex

Dear Teen-ager:

Girls need to "prove their love" through illicit sex relations like a moose needs a hat rack. Why not "prove your love" by sticking your head in the oven and turning on the gas? Or playing leap frog in the traffic? It's about as safe. Clear the cobwebs out of your head. Any fellow who asks you to "prove your love" is trying to take you for the biggest, most gullible fool who ever walked. That "proving" bit is one of the oldest and rottenest lines ever invented. Does he love you? It doesn't sound like it. Someone who loves you wants whatever is best for you. But now figure it out. He wants you to:

Commit an immoral act . . .

Surrender your virtue . . .

Throw away your self-respect . . .

Risk the loss of your precious reputation . . .

And risk getting into trouble.

Does that sound as though he wants the best for you? This is the laugh of the century. He wants what's best for him: he wants a thrill he can brag about at your expense . . . Love? Who's kidding whom?

A guy who loves a girl would sooner cut off his right arm than hurt her. In my opinion, this self-serving so-and-so has proved that he doesn't love you. The predictable aftermath of "proof" of this kind always finds Don Juan tiring of his sport.

That's when he drops you, picks up his line, and goes casting elsewhere for bigger and equally silly fish.

A Word of Encouragement

We've come to the end of discussing two subjects that I know you think about a great deal: dating and "shall we or shall we not go along with the crowd in having sex?" But I can't leave this section without a personal word to you.

First, I want to encourage you to trust Jesus to give you the mate best suited for you. I was absolutely ancient when I got married—thirty! The reason I tell you this is because I want you to know I understand what it is like to wait and wait to meet the right person. I also know what it is to be tempted to settle for someone who doesn't meet the standards we have set, simply because we're afraid that if we don't grab the chance we have, we may never get married. (Being unmarried is not the worst that could happen, though when we are young we often think it is.)

During my years of waiting I clung to a little verse that may help you:

> God knows, he loves, he cares.
> Nothing this truth can dim.
> He gives the very best to those
> Who leave the choice with him.

Recently I have been thinking back over the days when I was where you are now. I have recalled some of the fellows I dated. One committed suicide some years ago. Two have lived the type of life which would have left me feeling very frustrated. Another, I am told, isn't a Christian anymore. And there were others.

Then I think of the husband God finally gave me. He has enriched my life in every way, especially spiritually and intellectually, far beyond my dearest dreams. I can't thank the Lord enough for watching over and caring for me in this way.

So I plead with you to trust Jesus to provide the right mate for you. "Trust in the Lord with all your heart and lean not on your own understanding; in all your ways acknowledge him, and he will make your paths straight" (Prov. 3:5, 6, NIV). These verses sat on my desk for years as a reminder. And God was faithful to me, and He will be faithful to you too.

The second matter about which I want to say a word is purity. You will never, never, *never* regret keeping yourself pure for your one true love. God forgives us our sins, of course, but memories have a way of haunting us and surfacing at the most awkward times. When you and your true love finally meet in union, you don't want any memories of past experiences with others flitting through your mind. You will want to give yourself completely and without distraction to your spouse.

"But what do I do if I have already sinned?" you may ask.

Ah, yes. That is painful. What do you do?

You come to Jesus with your sin. You kneel before Him and ask Him to show you the meaning of sin and what your sin did to Him. Don't rush away. Let God speak to you. Let Him break your heart. Let the tears flow. Feel remorseful. This won't be something you work up by yourself, for that would have little meaning or value. Let the Holy Spirit work in your heart as you wait for Him.

Then ask Jesus to show you himself on the cross. Thank Him that, small as you are, you may take refuge in His greatness. Thank Him that no matter how terrible your sin, you may run to Him and His cross. Thank Him that though you have not loved Him as you ought, you may hide yourself in His forgiveness.

And then hear Him speak His sweet words of forgiveness to you. Open your heart and let the Holy Spirit pour into you that incredible peace that passes understanding. Become a new person. And having become a new person, walk out into the future with Jesus—in love with Him, delighting to do His will and eager to discover the surprises He has in store for you. God go with you, my friend.

If you need guidance to pray, use Psalm 51 as a model. The following verses will give you comfort and assurance of being forgiven by God: 1 John 1:9; Romans 8:1; John 6:37; Psalm 103:3, 4; Isaiah 43:1, 2, 5, 6, 25.

8 ❖ WHEN WILL I BE READY TO GET MARRIED?

Earlier in our discussion we said adolescence is a time of preparation for marriage. Let's talk about that some more now.

How can we get ready for marriage? When should we start dating? When should we start going steady? How do we know what is true love and what is infatuation? What responsibilities must we assume when we get married? How old do we have to be to assume those responsibilities? What does it mean to "leave" our parents? Why can't we live with parents after we are married? How long should we expect out parents to continue to support us? Why is liking ourselves such an important factor in a good marriage?

We'll now explore these and many more questions. This should be a fun chapter.

A Bible Study: What Does It Mean to Get Married?

Read Genesis 1:27 and 2:24 and then consider the following questions.

1. Some say sex is all right for engaged couples or couples who say they love each other. In these verses, what does God say two people who want to be married should do?

They should _____ their parents.

If the relationship between parents and children has been a good and loving one, is this easy to do? Why are tears sometimes shed at weddings?

Walter Trobisch, in *I Married You*, says, "Leaving is the price of happiness." He also says, "Parents can be compared to hens who hatch out duck eggs. After they are hatched, the duck-lings walk to the pond and swim away. But the hens cannot follow them. They stay on the banks of the pond and cackle."

What are some of the practical implications of this leaving? For example, with today's rents and housing costs being so high, some young married people feel they have to live with one of the parents for a while in order to save money for a down pay-ment. How can this be done if the person is supposed to "leave" his parents? In such a case, is it better to stay with the girl's or the boy's parents? What is the risk for the young couple? How can such an arrangement cause difficulty for parents?

What is the difference between "leaving" and abandoning?

What is the difference between viewing a woman as a mother-in-law and viewing her as a family member?

Which family is more likely to interfere in a young couple's marriage: the boy's family or the girl's family?

Sometimes young people leave their homes or parents in the wrong way. Can you explain how this happens?

2. Look at the second part of these verses: After a young couple leave their parents, they should _____ to one an-other.

What does the word "cleave" mean?

"Cleave" means to be closer to each other than any other person or any other thing. In the course of marriages, what things can become closer to either the husband or wife than each other?

Why do you suppose the word "cleave" is used instead of "love"?

If husband, wife and children are all glued together, what happens when divorce takes place? What feelings does this pro-duce?

3. When a young couple leave their parents and cleave to each other, what happens next?

What union does "one flesh" refer to?

What comes after the word "flesh" in Genesis 2:24? What is the significance of this? How does this offer comfort to couples who are not able to have children?

4. What rite or ceremony is observed publicly when young people want to leave their parents and be joined to each other?

5. After this ceremony is observed, what is permissible?

6. In our American culture we emphasize that there should be love between the man and woman before they think of mar-

riage. In many cultures, however, this is not true. I lived in India for seven years and many of the marriages there were arranged. When the Indians talked about the difference between Western and Eastern ways, some of them would quote a traditional proverb: "When you emphasize love before marriage," they would say, "it is like filling a pan with hot water and putting it on the stove, but the heat on the stove is only on low. The water cools off. We put a pan of cold water on the stove," they explained, "and even with the stove only on low, it slowly gets warm."

What do you understand by this saying?

In the musical play, *Fiddler on the Roof*, Tevye, the milkman, had his marriage with Golde arranged by his parents. But his teen-age children were taking matters into their own hands. They were falling in love and making their own decisions. Tevye watched this, puzzled.

One day he starts to talk with Golde about how different it had been for them. He hadn't even seen Golde until their wedding day. Both of them confess to each other how scared and shy and nervous they had been. But, Tevye reminds Golde, his parents had said the newlyweds would learn to love each other. Silence falls between the two.

Then shyly, Tevye asks Golde, "How is it, Golde—do you love me?"

Golde stares off into space. Can you guess her answer? Try to fill in the missing words:

"Do I love him?

For twenty-five years I've _____ with him.

_____ with him, _____ with him.

Twenty-five years my _____ is his.

If that's not _____ , what is?"[1]

How would you like to have your parents arrange your marriage? What would be the risk? What might be some good features?

More and more people in our Western culture try to enter marriage through sex. They don't wait for true love to grow. Do you agree or disagree with the following statements? Give reasons for your opinions.

    a. Love does not grow out of sex.

---

[1] *Fiddler on the Roof* by Joseph Stein, c. 1964 by Joseph Stein, Crown Publishing, Inc.

b. Love must grow into sex.[2]

According to the Bible, sexual intercourse means "becoming one flesh." In light of the biblical teaching, why is sex more than just experimentation or "the thing to do"?

---

[2]Questions from *I Married You* by Walter Trobisch, Harper & Row.

What Kind of a Person Do You Want to Marry?

What qualities of a person do you think contribute to a happy marriage and home? List them below.

At the same time ask your parents to list the qualities in their spouse that they have appreciated most.

When all of you have completed your lists, compare them. By the way, how many items on your list referred to the way a person looks? His clothes? Why do these things become less important as the years pass than they seem to be when we are young?

Could this list help you in any way when, in a few years, you will begin to think of going steady with one person?

What Do You Think of Yourself?

How would you complete the following statement: I feel loved and wanted and worthwhile when. . . .

In the space below, list the events and the things that make you feel loved and worthwhile. Now compare your list with the one on the next page.

I feel loved and wanted and worthwhile . . .

- When I have friends even if I don't like what I see in the mirror.
- When I can do something well.
- When I can forget myself and think of others.
- When I think about how much God loves me.
- When I know God has forgiven me.
- When someone compliments or thanks me.
- When I am obedient to my parents.
- When I do well in school.
- When I pray.
- When I take good care of my body.
- When I succeed.
- When I fail but don't get jealous or discouraged enough to give up.
- When I keep my room orderly and clean.
- When I learn some new skill.
- When I treat others with courtesy and respect.
- When I wear something I think is attractive.
- When I can lose graciously.
- When I say no to someone who wants me to do something I believe is wrong.
- When somebody tells me he is sure I can do something I haven't done before and am a little afraid to tackle.
- When I do something I was afraid to do (such as standing up in front of people and giving a report).
- When I say "I'm sorry" after I've done something wrong.

What did you mention that is not on this list? Did some of the items on this list remind you of things you had forgotten? Maybe you want to add some items to your list. Then take a moment to thank God for the things that you have mentioned. Thank Him that He has enabled you to do the things you are able to do and be the person you are.

Question: How do you think liking yourself and feeling good about yourself will affect your love and sex life?

What Responsibilities Are Involved in Marriage?

What are some of the responsibilities people assume or should assume when they get married? Make a list below of the responsibilities that come to your mind.

Ask your parents to make a similar list.

When all of you have completed your lists, compare them. If you are not working this exercise with your parents, you may want to compare your list with the list on the following page. What isn't on this list that you remembered on yours?

In order to have a happy marriage I want a mate who will . . .

1. Be able to help provide financially for the family.
2. Manage finances wisely.
3. Possess ability and willingness to care for a home.
4. Has ability or know-how to care for a car.
5. Has ability and willingness to care for a yard.
6. Is willing to share responsibilities in raising children if there are children.
7. Be able to and willing to cook appetizing and nourishing meals.
8. Be willing to live within a budget.
9. Make a commitment to care for his own health and the health of the family.
10. Make a commitment to give attention to the well-being of the family and develop and strengthen his own spiritual life and that of family members.

Now evaluate your list as to which items you think are the most important for your mate to fulfill in order that you may have a happy marriage. Number them 1, 2, 3, etc., in order of their importance. Which ones would you have difficulty fulfilling now? What will be needed in order for you to fulfill them well? Discuss this.

What's Marriage Like at Seventeen?

The following is a letter a 17-year-old girl sent to Ann Landers.

Let me tell you what it is like to be married at 17. It is like living in this dump on third floor. Your only window looks out on somebody else's third-floor dump.

It is like coming home so tired you feel nearly dead from standing all day at your checker's job in the supermarket. But you don't dare sit down because you might never get up. And there are so many things you have to do—cooking and washing and ironing. But you go through the motions and you hate your job.

You ask yourself, "Why don't you quit?" And you know why. Because there are grocery bills and drug bills and the rent to pay. And Jimmy's crummy little check from the lumberyard won't cover them. That's why.

Then you tell the sitter good-bye and you try to play with the baby until Jimmy comes home. Only sometimes you don't feel like it. But you do it anyway because you feel guilty about being away from her all day. Then you mix the formula and wash diapers and you hate doing it. And you wonder how long it will be before she can tell that you hate it. And wouldn't it be awful if she knew it already?

Then Jimmy doesn't come home again and you know he decided to go out with the boys again and do the things he should have gotten done before he married you.

So finally you eat the lousy meal by yourself and go to bed and cry your eyes out. When he does come home you can tell he's been drinking but you don't say a word because he hates to be told anything. So you try to go to sleep and dream about your parents and your brothers and sisters and the kids you knew at school. You think about the great meals your mother used to cook and how nice your room was at home.

Then you remember how she tried to talk you out of marrying so young and you got mad at her and called her a dried-up old woman and accused her of having forgotten what it was like to be in love.

You try to push the thoughts of other boys out of your mind but they keep coming back. Especially that certain boy who gave you your first kiss. He won the state science prize and is going to be a doctor.

You wonder how different your life would have been if you had gone to college. You have the feeling that Jimmy and the baby are all part of a bad dream. But you know it's no dream. It's for real. So you reach over to touch Jimmy, and he pushes you away and says something mean. So you cry yourself to sleep and wake up with a splitting headache. What a way to start another day of hard work.

If you meet anyone who thinks she knows what it is like to be married at 17, please give her my letter.

(Signed) Sorry[3]

Ann Landers added: "I could print a letter similar to this every day of the week, but what's the use? Are you listening out there? I hope so."

Habit Patterns

We all have habits. When we live with each other year after year and day after day, if our habits aren't alike, we may begin to annoy and irritate each other. Usually marriages are less stormy if both partners have at least some habits in common.

What habits would you like your partner to have? What habits do you have? Do you think any of them might be a source of annoyance to another person?

---

[3]Reprinted by permission from Ann Landers, News America Syndicate, and the *Forum Newspaper,* Fargo, North Dakota.

Read each of the following exercises and decide how you would act in each situation.

1. Don and Mary have been married six months. Mary is a very neat person, but Don leaves his clothes lying on the floor, which annoys Mary. How can Don and Mary solve this problem? You suggest some solutions first. Then ask your parents how they would solve this problem.

2. Janelle likes to stay up late and sleep in, because she doesn't have to be at her job until 9 o'clock. Mark, on the other hand, has to commute a long way to work. He has to rise at 5:00 a.m. At night he is tired and wants to go to bed at 9 p.m. They don't see each other in the morning, and have little time together in the evening. What can Janelle and Mark do so they have some time together?

3. During Karen's childhood her mother worked, so Karen practically grew up on fast foods and convenience foods. She still likes them and doesn't like to cook. Terry's mother, on the other hand, always prepared complete home-cooked dinners. Terry prefers them. How can Terry and Karen work this out satisfactorily?

4. Paul loves to watch Saturday football and baseball games on TV, but Saturday is the one day when Barbara and Paul are completely free to do something together. Barbara wants to go places and do things. Paul wants to stay home and watch the games. How can Paul and Barbara solve this?

5. Jason and Christi have been married about six months. They live in a small apartment. Jason is hooked on watching sports on TV whenever there is a game, but the apartment is so small Christi doesn't know where to go while the TV is on. It is bugging her more and more. What can the two do?

Questions Kids Ask

1. *I'm 17. I'll be 18 next spring when I graduate from high school. I've just met this neat new guy at school, and we both love each other. We want to be married next spring. My parents say I have to wait at least two years. Why do they think it's so necessary to wait? We know we're in love and want to get married.*

Quite likely your parents are concerned because they know that 50% of all teen-age marriages end in divorce. One reason this happens is because kids confuse infatuation with love. How can you distinguish between the two?

Infatuation, that glorious, giddy feeling, is first of all self-centered. When you are infatuated, you are thinking chiefly about how excited you are, and how loved you feel. True love is concerned with the happiness and well-being of the other person.

Second, the romantic feelings of infatuation are like the rushing waters of a mountain brook in spring. The trouble is, when the hot summer comes, the brook runs dry. In the same way, the "high" feelings of infatuation never last. Even in good solid marriages romantic feelings don't persist all the time. There may be stretches when one doesn't feel particularly in love with the other. But in spite of that you continue to live with and accept the other person. Even if the other one becomes so grumpy, irritable, out-of-sorts, lazy or short-tempered that it is difficult to like him or her, still you stick with your mate. That's love. Infatuation gives up.

One of the most effective tests of a relationship is *time*. How much time? The younger you are, the longer the time should be. If you are still in your teens, I'd say two years at least. After all, marriage should be for keeps, for life.

Six or seven years from now you'll be surprised at how greatly what attracts you to a person has changed from what it is now. For example, in the survey of 3,000 girls from 13–19 years of age that *Seventeen* magazine conducted some time ago, here is what the girls listed as attracting them to fellows:

Looks—46.5%
Friendliness—38.8%
Sense of humor—10.1%
Personality—5.3%
Intelligence—5.5%

Does that sound familiar?

Interestingly, if you were to ask women 25–30 years of age the same question, the list would probably be reversed completely, with intelligence, personality and sense of humor rated high and looks rated very low.

Some single women in their late twenties were discussing men, and one said, "If Bob weren't married to Tammy,[4] I'd do anything I could to marry him."

This attractive young woman was talking about a man who is short, overweight, and balding. So why did he seem so won-

---

[4]Not their real names.

derful? He cared about people and was fun to be with. Believe me, the older you get, the more your values will change!

This is why teen-agers wishing to marry need to make the decision slowly, carefully and prayerfully. Then their relationship should be tested by a period of engagement. It's better to break an engagement than go through a divorce.

2. *Do you believe God has chosen one particular person for me to marry?*

I believe we should pray for God's guidance and can be confident He will help us. But God has given us minds to think and wills to choose, and He expects us to use both wisely. Though some people testify God gave them a direct command in a dream or vision to marry someone whom they did not know well or love, this is certainly not the usual way in which God guides.

3. *Our neighbor's little girl got spinal meningitis and now is blind and doesn't seem able to think. Mom says the girl's parents have been fighting so much Mom's afraid the marriage will break up. What's wrong. Didn't they really ever love each other? Doesn't true love survive everything?*

Love can survive very difficult situations such as the one you described, but sometimes it doesn't. Why? Because love is fragile and needs careful handling. Love is a living thing, and all living things need to be nourished and tended if they are going to survive. Couples have to work extra hard to keep their love healthy when they run into trouble of any kind. They also need other friends who will help them understand themselves and their reactions, friends who will shoulder their problems with them. It is difficult for a couple to face hard problems on their own.

4. *Why can't people just live together without getting married? Why is getting married important or necessary?*

Marriage, first of all, is a special relationship of love between two people. It is used in the Bible to describe the relationship God has with His people. The book of Hosea refers to this often, and the Apostle Paul also writes of this in Ephesians 5:25–32.

Marriage also carries the meaning of two people covenanting to be true to each other until death separates them. Jesus referred to this when He said, " 'Haven't you read,' he replied, 'that at the beginning the Creator "made them male and female," ' and said, "For this reason a man will leave his father and mother and be united to his wife, and the two will become one flesh"? So they are no longer two, but one. Therefore what God has joined together, let man not separate' " (Matt. 19:4–6, NIV).

The sanctity, that is, the specialness or the uniqueness of marriage, is referred to in Hebrews 13:4: "Marriage should be honored by all, and the marriage bed kept pure, for God will judge the adulterer and all the sexually immoral" (NIV). Marriage, this verse declares, is good and honorable, to be respected by all. Sex is an integral part of marriage. People are not to engage in sex unless married, and married people should not have sex with anyone except the one to whom they are married.

Society or the state recognizes people as being married when they have applied for a license to be married and then later have entered into a legal contract by promising to be faithful to each other in the presence of a clergyman or someone authorized by the government to marry people. This helps provide a safeguard against unwise marriages and unfaithfulness in marriage. Christians should therefore have their marriage covenants certified by a legal contract as well as seek the blessing of the church by a public ceremony.

Can This Marriage Survive?

Fred and Mary have been married six months. They came from different home backgrounds. Whenever they begin to quarrel Fred says, "Your mother never taught you how to cook."

Mary says, "Your parents are stuffy. They don't know how to have a good time."

Fred says, "Their house is always a mess."

Mary says, "Your folks have weird ideas about sex."

Fred says, "Your folks never did have any time for God and the church."

Mary says, "Your parents had more time for church than they did for you kids. What kind of religion is that?"

Where will this kind of talk get Fred and Mary?

What do their remarks tell us about the relationship they had before they were married?

Do you think their marriage can survive?

What do Fred and Mary need to do?[5]

---

[5]For more help on how to live in harmony read *Telling Each Other the Truth,* William Backus (Minneapolis: Bethany House Publishers, 1985).

9 ❖ CONTRACEPTIVES: BLESSING OR DISGUISED DISASTER?

If we don't believe in having sex outside of marriage, why should we talk about contraceptives at all? For a number of reasons, but mainly because teen-agers have a lot of misinformation about contraceptives. Because of this some are lulled into believing they aren't taking chances—when they are. Contraceptives, even when used correctly, are not 100% effective.

The information given here is *not* to lull you into thinking that pre-marital sex is all right. It isn't.

There are two main reasons for including this chapter. First of all, you need to know the facts when your friends say things on this subject that are untrue and even dangerous. Second, young people need *accurate* information. For example, you may have heard that withdrawal is safe. It isn't. You may think that an intrauterine device is the answer, but not know that in some cases it causes infections, which, in turn, cause sterility. Then years later after you have married and *want* children, you might be unable to have them.

Being misinformed is like lighting a match close to an open gasoline tank. The whole thing could explode in your face.

Another reason you need to know something about contraceptives is that after you get married, you probably will want to decide how many children you want and how you would like to space them. That will be the *right* time for you to use contraceptives. But again you need to know what the different contraceptives are, how safe they are, what complications can result from using them, etc.

We aren't going to give detailed information in this book,

however, so when you are ready for marriage, you will want to study this subject more carefully and consult with your doctor, and possibly your pastor. But let's learn a few basic facts now.

Questions Kids Ask About Contraception

1. *If the fellow practices withdrawal, that is, taking out his penis before reaching orgasm, can't he be sure the girl won't get pregnant?*

No. Some of the semen can escape before orgasm takes place. Remember that hundreds of millions of little cells are ready to go every time one gets sexually aroused. There's no way to be sure you've controlled them all by practicing withdrawal. Many of them can easily escape before orgasm.

2. *Isn't it true that there are certain days in a girl's menstrual cycle when she won't get pregnant?*

The "safe" period in a woman's cycle is usually from the 1st to the 10th day of her cycle and from the 19th through the 28th day of her cycle. This form of contraception is sometimes called the "rhythm method." Some girls, however, do not have regular cycles, which makes it difficult to determine exactly which are the "safe" days. There are books which describe the techniques to determine "safe" days.

3. *If I drink a lot of alcohol before I have sex, won't the sperm be so drunk they can't find the egg?*

The alcohol won't affect the sperm at all. Besides, the Bible has a great deal to say about drunkenness.

4. *If a person doesn't experience orgasm, can't she be sure she won't get pregnant?*

There is no relationship at all between the two. A girl may not experience an orgasm and still get pregnant.

5. *If I squirt liquid into my vagina or take a douche after having sex, can't I be sure that I won't get pregnant?*

Neither will do you one speck of good as far as preventing pregnancy.

6. *If a girl urinates right after sex, won't she get rid of the boy's sperm?*

The urethra, the tube through which you urinate, is completely separate from the organs of your body involved in sex. Urinating will do absolutely no good at all. A boy's sperm enter a girl's vagina, pass through the uterus, and continue on up into the Fallopian tubes. This area is completely separate from the urethra.

7. *If a boy wraps Saran Wrap around his penis, won't that keep sperm from entering the girl's vagina?*

No. The only reasonably safe contraceptive of this type is the condom, a rubber "balloon" which fits over the penis. But the condom must be new and undamaged, and must be used properly according to instructions. The condom may prevent conception, but Saran Wrap is worse than useless. A fellow who suggests that route is simply trying to con the girl into satisfying his own sexual needs—it certainly won't satisfy hers! A "Saran Wrap" attitude about sex has no understanding of *mutual* love and pleasure in marriage.

8. *If a couple has sex regularly for a year, what are the chances that she will get pregnant?*

If no contraceptives are used, 90 out of 100 women will get pregnant within a year's time. Using withdrawal, 20–25 out of 100 will get pregnant. Using the rhythm method, 20–25 will conceive, and the number will be the same for those who use contraceptive foam properly. Of those who use the diaphragm (a rubber barrier placed in the vagina) with sperm-killing jelly, 15–20 out of 100 will conceive. When the male uses the condom and uses it exactly according to directions, about 5–15 women out of 100 will get pregnant. Some say the pill, if used properly, is virtually 100% effective and that it is very effective even if an occasional pill is missed. Others say that 5 to 10 out of every 100 still will get pregnant. Only 5 out of 100 using the intra-uterine device will conceive, but there are dangers with this device, and a doctor must insert it. Sometimes the uterus will spontaneously reject it and expel it.

As you can see, no contraceptives are 100% effective in preventing conception. So the only way to be sure of avoiding pregnancy before marriage is to avoid having sex. That's 100% effective. And that, after all, is God's plan.

How Much Do you Know About Contraceptives?

(Match the correct term with the definition at the right. Answers are on the next page.)

_____ 1. A chemical that causes chemical changes in a woman's body to stop her from ovulating.

_____ 2. A round rubber cap a woman places in the vagina before she has intercourse.

_____ 3. A thin finger-like rubber device that a man fits over his erect penis before intercourse.

_____ 4. Foams, cream or jellies placed in the woman's vagina to kill sperm.

_____ 5. A plastic ring, coil or loop inserted in the uterus by a doctor.

_____ 6. The method whereby a couple has intercourse only during the so-called "safe" period.

_____ 7. The man pulls his penis out before ejaculation of the semen takes place.

_____ 8. A short section of each vas deferens is cut and the ends tied.

_____ 9. Fallopian tubes are cut and tied.

_____ 10. Refraining from sexual intercourse.

a. diaphragm
b. withdrawal
c. intrauterine devices
d. rhythm method
e. condom
f. the pill
g. abstinence
h. spermicides
i. vasectomy
j. tubal ligation

Answers to How Much Do You Know About Contraceptives?

1. *(f) The pill.* When a woman does not ovulate, this means no egg is released. If there is no egg with which the sperm can unite, pregnancy cannot take place.

The pill is used in two ways. In the first case one pill is taken for three weeks, beginning on the fifth day after menstruation begins. Then the pills are stopped for one week during which a menstrual period of sorts takes place. In the other case a pill is taken every day without a seven-day break during the 28-day cycle.

The pill is considered physically safe when prescribed by a physician for a healthy young woman. After the age of 35, and especially if the woman smokes, there are health risks involved. The chief concern is that blood clots might develop which, if they travel to the lung, brain or heart, can be fatal. Pill users also have been found three times as likely to have heart attacks. There also seem to be increased vaginal discharge, increased incidence of gallbladder disease and hypertension, and various vitamin deficiencies among pill users. In some cases brown splotches appear on the skin. Pill users also appear to be more susceptible to diabetes and liver tumors.

2. *(a) Diaphragm.* The cap is about two to three inches in diameter. A doctor insures that it fits properly, writes a prescription for it, and shows the woman how to insert it. The diaphragm is used with a spermicidal jelly. The diaphragm holds the spermicide in place over the cervix so that the spermicide can work effectively, but without the spermicide the diaphragm is useless.

3. *(e) Condom.* The condom, which prevents the sperm from escaping to the vagina, is available without prescription. To be effective it must be new and must be used exactly according to the manufacturer's instructions. If a condom is not used properly, it is unreliable. If used properly with a spermicide it is one of the most effective.

4. *(h) Spermicides.* While not as effective as the pill or the IUD, spermicides are used by many women successfully. They are available in drugstores without prescription. They have a failure rate of between 20 and 25%.

5. *(c) Intrauterine devices.* The intrauterine devices (IUD) work by causing a local inflammation that prevents the implantation of the fertilized egg. It is relatively inexpensive to

use. Once a doctor inserts the device nothing more needs to be done except for the woman to see the doctor periodically to check for complications. Between 5 and 20% of the women spontaneously expel the device, however. Some women experience excessive menstrual bleeding, spotting between periods, cramping and lower back pain. There is also danger of infection. If the infection persists, it can cause sterility, illness and even death. Once in a while, though rarely, the wall of the uterus is perforated when the IUD is inserted, and hemorrhaging, even to the point of death, may result. (A manufacturer lost a multi-million-dollar suit because of the injuries blamed on its IUD.) If a pregnancy should occur when the IUD is in place, in 50% of the cases a miscarriage occurs. If a doctor doesn't remove the IUD immediately, blood poisoning and infection may result. Some women have died.

Because the IUD causes a fertilized egg to be rejected, in a sense it aborts the embryo. Many people therefore believe it is morally wrong to use the IUD as a contraceptive device.

6. *(d) Rhythm method.* The problem with this method is that the medical world has not been able to find an easy and accurate way of telling when ovulation occurs. The "safe" period for a woman usually is from the 1st to the 10th day of her cycle, and from the 19th through the 28th day of her cycle, but a woman's cycle may not always be regular.

There are, however, no health risks with this method, and because of the considerable risks involved with many other contraceptives, researchers are continuing to seek ways for determining accurately when ovulation is taking place.

The rhythm method is also referred to as "natural family planning." Another method listed under "natural family planning" is the symptothermal technique. It is necessary for both husband and wife to study the method and both of them must follow the directions without fail. It requires the woman to record and graph her temperature each morning, and to check daily the kind of mucus discharged from her vagina. But this plan also means that couples cannot enjoy sex for rather long periods each month. That can be hard. But advocates of the method claim it is extremely effective—if followed faithfully. And there are no health risks involved.

7. *(b) Withdrawal.* This is an old method. The problem with it is the man may not withdraw quickly enough or some semen may escape even before ejaculation. The need to withdraw brings

a certain amount of tension into the sexual act which can hinder the couple's full enjoyment of intercourse. Withdrawal is not reliable, but it probably prevents some pregnancies.

8. *(i) Vasectomy.* This is used by some couples who want no more children. Cutting and tying the vas deferens of the man prevents the semen from passing along the tube and out the penis to the woman's body. Instead, the body absorbs the sperm. It is a minor, easy, and relatively inexpensive operation to perform on a man who is sure he no longer wants to have children.

9. *(j) Tubal ligation.* In this surgical operation on a woman, the Fallopian tubes are cut so the egg cells cannot pass from the ovaries to the uterus. The surgery must be performed in the hospital. The surgeon makes a small incision in the navel, inserts a tiny telescope through which he can see what he is doing. He then inserts an electric cauterizer to burn out a small section of each tube and seal it closed, which is considered to be permanent. Usually the patient does not even need to stay overnight in the hospital. There also are other methods of performing tubal ligation.

10. *(g) Abstinence.* While this may be practiced for short periods, for example during times of illness or recuperation, it is an unnatural, abnormal procedure for a married couple to practice regularly. Sex binds a couple together, alleviates tension, and is a means of expressing love. To deny one's mate does not contribute to a happy marriage. Read the Apostle Paul's advice in 1 Corinthians 7:2–6.

In addition to the methods of contraception mentioned above, a sponge soaked in spermicide and placed deep in the vagina is being used by some. The FDA has approved this as being almost 85% dependable, but the method is very new and needs more testing.

Some Christians firmly believe that any form of artificial contraception is wrong. They therefore advocate only natural means such as withdrawal or some form of the rhythm method. We should respect their beliefs and come to a clear conclusion about what method God would have us use when we are married.

For youth who are not married the simplest and best and happiest way to avoid an unwanted pregnancy is to say a firm no. In fact, "NO" buttons are available from a group in Denver (P.O. Box 6480, Denver, CO. 80206). If you say no, you don't have to worry about which contraceptives to use, how to use them or what risks are involved. So isn't saying no both safest and easiest?

Abortion, as it is most frequently practiced, is also a form of contraceptive. Let's consider that subject next.

Twenty Questions About Abortion

1. *My girlfriend at school said her mother had a miscarriage. What does that mean?*

Your friend's mother was pregnant, but she wasn't able to carry her baby full term. If the muscles of the uterus contract and force out the fetus before it is four months old, this is referred to by lay people as miscarriage. Medical people refer to miscarriage as "spontaneous abortion." No one knows for sure why spontaneous abortions occur. There probably are many reasons, and someday doctors may discover them.

2. *What is the difference between a spontaneous abortion and an induced abortion?*

In a spontaneous abortion the fetus is expelled from the mother's uterus without the mother doing anything. It just happens. Induced abortion means the fetus, the placenta and the tissue is purposely removed from the uterus of the mother. There are five methods by which this is done.

Sometimes it is done surgically. The mother is given an anaesthesia and a surgeon removes with an instrument the fetus, placenta and tissue. This operation is called a D and C, or *Dilation and Curettage*. Sometimes when a mother has had a miscarriage, some of the tissue might be left inside the uterus. This causes bleeding, and the mother then has to have a D and C to get her uterus clean and stop the bleeding.

Another surgical procedure is called *Dilation and Evacuation* (D and E). It is also known as "vacuum suction" and "vacuum curettage." The method was introduced in China in 1958 and in the U.S. in the mid-1960s.

A local anaesthetic is given, usually in a doctor's office. The physician dilates the cervix by inserting larger and larger rod-shaped instruments; he finally inserts a rigid metal or plastic hollow instrument connected to a long tube which is attached to an electrical or mechanical pump. The fetus is ripped apart by the suction action and suctioned out. The procedure takes about ten minutes.

Sometimes a girl may use the *morning-after pill* if she has had intercourse without using a contraceptive. The girl takes two pills a day for five days and must start no later than three days after the sexual act. The pill contains a huge dose of a synthetic estrogen (DES) made from coal tar. It is thought the pill prevents a fertilized egg from burrowing in the soft, cushiony walls of the uterus. But side effects such as nausea and vomiting are frequent. Also the use of DES has been linked to much higher than normal rates of vaginal and cervical cancer.

Another procedure, used after a girl has been pregnant sixteen weeks, is called the *saline abortion.* A long needle is inserted into the sac containing amniotic fluid in which the baby floats. Through the needle some of the amniotic fluid is drawn out and replaced with a solution of concentrated salt. The salt solution goes into the lungs and digestive tract of the fetus. It also burns off the outer layer of skin of the fetus. It usually takes an hour before the life of the baby comes to an end. The mother goes into labor about a day later, and she gives birth to a dead baby—usually. A few of these babies have been born alive.

The fourth technique is called a *hysterotomy* and is sometimes used, though actually very rarely, if the pregnancy has continued 13 weeks or more. An incision is made in the abdomen and uterus, and the fetus and placenta are removed. This is a surgical operation. The baby is left to die on its own. Babies removed at this stage and in this way are very small but some have been known to move arms and legs, gasp a few breaths and appear to make efforts to cry.

The fifth method is called *prostaglandin chemical abortion.* A compound causes the muscles to contract and push out the baby. Some babies aborted in this way have been born alive.

3. *We had an argument in school. I said only doctors can perform abortions. One of the girls said she knows of people who have gone to abortion clinics where there is no doctor. Does that happen?*

The majority of abortions are performed in hospitals by qualified doctors. Some clinics, however, have been found to be operating without licenses and under unsanitary conditions which further increase risks for the mother. The increasing number of cases of infection, hemorrhaging, perforated uteri and even death betray the risks in any abortion, risks that are

severely compounded when an abortion is performed by an unqualified person.

4. *Our teacher said legalizing abortions has made them safer,
that years ago poor women used to go wherever they could for
help and they often died. Is this true?*

It is true that in the past thousands of women, many of them
poor and left to care for their children alone, went to unqualified
people to get an abortion because the law did not allow a physician to conduct one. These women suffered. Today the laws
have changed. Women can get abortions in most hospitals.

But unfortunately this has not reduced the number of illegal abortions. Instead, in Scandinavia, Hungary, East Ger-
many and England criminal abortions have increased since
abortions became legal. Official sources from New York and
Colorado have reported the same trend in their states. Making
abortion legal, therefore, has not lessened the number of illegal
abortions performed, but rather the numbers have increased.

5. *My teacher says only Catholics are against abortion. Is that
true?*

No, and anybody reading the news and listening to televi-
sion knows that is not true. But even before we began to see
public action against abortion taken by Christian groups, most
major Protestant theologians had opposed it. Their names may
not be familiar to you: Calvin, Ramsey, Barth, Thielecke, Bon-
hoeffer and many others. All of them were Protestants.

6. *Does a baby have a soul from the time it is conceived?*

Psalm 139:13–16 uses the Hebrew word for fetus to indicate
that this is so. Some say the fetus doesn't have a soul until it
is capable of life outside the mother, and they refer to Exodus
21:22, 23. However, there is much disagreement as to whether
this passage refers to the aborting of a child or the premature
live birth of a child, and the text is not often referred to anymore.

Although the passage in Psalm 139 is the only one where
the actual word "fetus" is used, there are many other references
to God's concern for the unborn child.

"Before I formed you in the womb I knew you, before you
were born I set you apart; I appointed you as a prophet to the
nations" (Jer. 1:5, NIV).

"Your hands made me and formed me. . . (Ps. 119:73, NIV).

"For you created my inmost being; you knit me together in my mother's womb. I praise you because I am fearfully and wonderfully made; your works are wonderful, I know that full well. My frame was not hidden from you when I was made in the secret place. When I was woven together in the depths of the earth, your eyes saw my unformed body. All the days ordained for me were written in your book before one of them came to be. How precious to me are your thoughts, O God! How vast is the sum of them!" (Ps. 139:13–17, NIV).

"Did not he who made me in the womb make them? Did not the same one form us both within our mothers?" (Job 31:15, NIV).

"Did you not . . . clothe me with skin and flesh and knit me together with bones and sinews? You gave me life and showed me kindness, and in your providence watched over my spirit" (Job 10:10–12, NIV).

All the person's potential, his sex, appearance, color of hair and eyes, height, physique, capacity for intelligent learning, special talents and personality characteristics, are present in the fetus. Can we therefore believe that God would leave out the most important thing of all, the soul? How can it be right for us to destroy all this?

Also, while it is true that the fetus is only about a half-inch long when it is a month old, its inner ear and eye structure already are formed, its heart is beating, its brain is growing and its circulatory system, liver and kidneys are all present. How then can we refer to such complexity as a mere clump of tissue? It is too immature to live outside the mother, but does that mean it does not have life?

Some medical researchers also believe the time is near when babies at a much earlier stage of development will be able to be kept alive outside of the mother. When this happens undoubtedly this will change many laws, and people's opinions and beliefs, as to whether or not a fetus is a whole person.

7. *There's this girl at school who had an abortion. Afterward she played real cool about it, even bragged about it. But one day she started talking to me about it and broke down and cried and cried.*

I can understand that. Many girls and women go through severe emotional struggles after having an abortion. They feel sad and guilty and hate themselves. God is always ready to forgive us when we come to Him confessing our sin (1 John 1:9), but many who have gone through something as emotional as an abortion have trouble receiving God's forgiveness.

It is even more serious when a girl can talk herself into believing "it's nothing." She can become so deaf to the voice of the Holy Spirit that she can't hear Him speaking to her at other times also.

If we have given our hearts and lives to Jesus, we belong to Him. If we belong to Him, then it follows that we listen to Him and obey Him. Others may do differently, but we cannot answer for them. We can and must answer for ourselves and our final answer will be made to God. That is a very sobering thought, isn't it?

In addition to suffering emotionally, some women suffer physically as the result of an abortion. The next time they get pregnant after having had an abortion, they run a greater risk of miscarriage or premature birth, and this is even more true if the mother is a teen-ager.

We need to offer all the love, support and help we can to those who are suffering because they had an abortion. Jesus cares. He wants them restored. He wants to help, to bring peace and comfort.

8. *One of the girls at school didn't have an abortion. She had her baby, and her parents are raising the little boy. Do you think this is a good idea?*

It is one alternative to abortion. I know of one instance where so far it is working out well. What the outcome will be in the years to come remains to be seen.

9. *Grandma says if a girl gets pregnant she should get married to the boy who made her pregnant. What do you think about that?*

Years ago when a girl became pregnant her parents usually insisted that the girl and boy get married. That is not necessarily a wise decision. Sometimes a girl gets pregnant by a boy whom she does not know well or love. Should she be forced to marry him? I would guess that the marriage very likely will not be happy and may not even last.

Young people's ideas change greatly between the mid-teens and 30. A girl may be attracted to one type of boy in her teens, but by the time she is in her twenties she may wonder what she ever saw in that fellow. Teen-age marriages are risky. Most teen-agers are not mature enough to be married.

10. *A girl at school who's 16 says she's going to keep her baby. How will she be able to do that?*

Usually a girl who makes this decision needs help in order to do this. Sometimes her family will help. Sometimes this works out happily, but sometimes it doesn't. Martha Zimmerman, in her book *Should I Keep My Baby?,*[1] lists 23 questions a girl should ask herself before deciding to keep her baby. Some of the questions she asks are:

- Have I ever cared for a child for 24 hours? A weekend? A week?
- How do I act when I am angry or upset?
- Do I get along with my parents?
- Would a child right now change my educational plans?
- Could I support a child financially?
- Would I be willing to give up the freedom to do what I want to do when I want to do it?
- Am I willing to give the next 18 years or more of my life to love and be responsible for my child, and to place concern for his or her well-being above my own?

11. *We were talking about all this the other night, and my mom said she thought placing the child for adoption was the best solution. Do you think adopted kids are happy?*

You almost are asking two questions. Let's try to answer your last question first—by asking another question: Do you think all kids born naturally into families are happy? Some adopted kids are very happy, some are middlin' happy, some are unhappy—just as other kids are. Many factors play a part in whether or not we are happy. Adoption is only one factor.

Now as to your question about whether or not adoption is a good solution for an unmarried mother: Offering a child for adoption can be an act of unselfish love both toward the child and toward the parents who adopt the child. Many married couples who cannot have children are overjoyed to get a baby and can provide well in every way for the child. But before they are given a child, they are interviewed and examined carefully. Their ages, personalities, ability to express love, financial status, health and religious faith are all thoughtfully considered.

---

[1]Martha Zimmerman, *Should I Keep My Baby?* (Minneapolis: Bethany House Publishers, 1983), pp. 44–45.

New parents of adoptive children are screened carefully to insure, as far as possible, the happiness of the child.

Adoption can be arranged either through an agency or by private placement. State laws govern the procedures.

12. *Isn't it hard for a girl to give up her baby?*

Without question most girls feel sad and experience a sense of loss. A few wonder afterward if they made the right choices. Some older women who had a baby in their teens and placed it for adoption confess they often wonder where their child is. They think about their child especially on birthdays or Mother's Day. Some say they wonder if their child is angry with them for what they did. Giving up a little life you've carried for nine months never is easy.

Without question, it's best, isn't it, not to be in the position of wondering what to do with a pregnancy? For a very few women this may not be possible. These women need all the help we can give them in every way. But most unmarried teen-agers can prevent it from happening simply by saying no.

13. *A woman on our street was raped when she was walking in the park one night. Now she's pregnant. Isn't it okay if she has an abortion?*

As Christians we always should be working for healing and preserving human life. We believe that people have a right to live and that right should take precedence over the comfort and convenience of others. In other words, it is wrong to end life just because people want their lives to be easier.

Some people believe there are certain instances when abortion may be considered permissible. For example, if a fetus is missing a brain or has too small a brain to enable the life to function as a person they consider it inhumane to expect a mother to care for such a life. In an interview in 1985, Billy Graham suggested pregnancies that result because of incest or rape also could be terminated by abortion. He admitted, however, he had second thoughts about the latter after he learned the late Ethel Waters, a famous gospel singer, was born out of such a situation.

Physician Thomas Elkins, an obstetrician/gynecologist at the University of Tennessee Medical Center, a Christian and the father of a Down's syndrome child, stated in an interview published in *Christianity Today*, "I couldn't do an abortion unless I thought the life of the mother was going to be lost. . . .

People ask me about rape and incest. I have trouble with it. Is the functional life of a mother going to be lost by giving birth to a child out of rape or incest? But to force a mother to carry a fetus without a brain is almost inhuman."

In the same issue of that magazine Lewis B. Smedes, professor of theology and ethics at Fuller Theological Seminary, said, "I believe that in our decision making we must have a passion for life, but a compassion for the living. There is a need for line drawing, but life does not allow us to draw permanent lines for every situation. We must allow for the exercise of what Saint Paul called 'spiritual understanding and wisdom' in those cases where sad and tragic decisions must be made."[2]

Mother Teresa of India has been one of the most outspoken advocates of the right of a child to live. When she accepted the Nobel Peace Prize in 1979, Mother Teresa said, "To me the nations that have legalized abortion are the poorest nations. They are afraid of the unborn child and the child must die." Later, when speaking to some women in New Delhi, she said, "If a mother can destroy her child, then how can you stop people from killing one another? . . . In all the suffering I see I ask myself why. The answer is that we are destroying the child. The life God has created, we kill. . . . We have been created in love. I beg you to use that power."

A short while later, speaking at Marquette University, she said: "And today, no one is more unwanted, no one is more unloved than the little unborn child. And yet, we know it was the little unborn child that recognized the presence of Christ when Mary came to Elizabeth. The little one in the womb of Elizabeth leaped with joy at the presence of Christ. And today, let us all unite to pray that in this beautiful country, we will make sure that we want the child . . . and that we will not allow a single child, a single unborn child, to feel unwanted, unloved, uncared for. For me, abortion is the greatest poverty that the nation can have, can experience."

Referring to abortion in America she said, "If you don't want that little child, that unborn child, give him to me. I want him."

It should also be pointed out in connection with pregnancies resulting from rape, as Mary Schott Ward, coordinator of the National Organization for Women's Committee on Rape, has noted, that pregnancy resulting from rape is rare. In a study

---

[2]*Christianity Today,* Jan. 18, 1985.

in Buffalo, New York, there hasn't been a confirmed pregnancy due to rape in over thirty years. Over a ten-year period in the Minneapolis/St. Paul metropolitan area, there were over 3,500 rapes reported with zero cases of pregnancy.

How can this be? Studies have shown that rapists very often are infertile or have had vasectomies, so they cannot get a woman pregnant. Many women, especially most married women, also are using some contraceptive method at the time of rape. Also, the chances of the rape occurring exactly at the time of a woman's ovulation are rare. And, mysteriously, it appears that the shock a woman experiences at a time of rape actually prevents the woman from ovulating, even though under normal circumstances she would do so.

It also should be stated that if a victim of a rape seeks medical help within a few hours following the rape, pregnancy often can be prevented.

This question needs to be asked too: Will having an abortion add to the mental and emotional distress of the raped woman? The wronged woman needs all the loving help we can give her. As Christians we can testify that we have seen God take very tragic happenings and turn them into something beautiful. His power to redeem is unlimited.

Have we ever tested to the fullest His ability to heal our hurts and to change our emotions from painful ones to ones of peace and trust? He stands ready to enable us always to forgive and, when needed, to love and care for the innocent life that may have been conceived in us even against our will. God also can give us courage and faith to respond to a challenge too big for us to meet in our own strength. God is faithful to His promises, and He will never let us down. I want to say it again: As we face difficult problems we must never limit ourselves to our poor human resources but focus instead on Jesus our Redeemer, and the Holy Spirit our Enabler.

14. *My mother says since contraceptives have become easily available to teen-agers and since abortions were legalized, the number of teen-agers becoming pregnant has increased greatly. Is this really so?*

Some claim that when and if contraceptives are easily available fewer pregnancies will result. Surveys have disproved this, however. Instead, more and more teen-agers have become sexually active. Many believe this has resulted because the kids are led to believe that little risk of pregnancy is involved if they use contraceptives. Contraceptives, however, are not 100% effective. Surveys have shown that regular users of contraceptives accounted for 14% of all premarital teen-age pregnancies in 1979, and far more than one-sixth of all unintended pregnancies. Almost one-third (31.5%) of the unintended pregnancies among metropolitan teen-agers in 1979 occurred while a contraceptive method was in use. And nearly half of the pregnancies occurred among young women who had used contraceptives at some time.

And in a survey Professors John F. Kantner and Melvin Zelnik of Johns Hopkins University took of teen-age sexual activity in the U.S. in 1979, it was shown that during the first eight years of a family planning program called Title X, the percentage of teen-agers experiencing a premarital pregnancy almost doubled.

I wonder, as you talk with your peers and friends at school, what your observations are. Do you think there would be as many youth participating in premarital sex if there were no contraceptives available and if abortion was not an option?

15. *One of my teachers said the U.S. has been slow in offering help to teen-agers who wanted information and help with their sexual lives. She said England offered this kind of help 25 years ago. Is she correct?*

In the 1960s England adopted a liberal contraceptive policy for teen-agers. Dr. Margaret White pointed out in her speech to the Human Life Convention in Seattle, however, that England resultantly experienced a sharp increase in venereal diseases, teen-age pregnancies and abortions. She gave two reasons for this: the implicit approval of premarital intercourse among teen-agers by society and the irresponsibility of teen-agers to use contraceptives in a disciplined, regular manner.

16. *I think educating kids about contraceptives is a good deal. It prevents pregnancies—and isn't that what we want to do? If kids don't get pregnant, they don't have to worry about the abortion problem.*

In the first place, let us make sure that educating about contraceptives really prevents pregnancies, shall we? From the results of actual surveys conducted, Dr. Michael Swartz and Dr. James H. Ford declare that birth control programs have not reduced the number of teen-age pregnancies. Instead, they insist, the programs have caused the problem to grow so that it is becoming a major social crisis.

They believe this has happened because youth have been encouraged to use birth control techniques. In addition they have been given the back-up promise that if contraceptives fail and a pregnancy results, the girl always can get an abortion.

Also, with clinics readily offering confidential help to teen-agers and stressing that youth need feel no guilt because of their action, more and more teen-agers are taking chances by having sex more frequently.[3]

17. *But I can't understand why this should be the case.*

In the first place, a sudden and drastic change in attitudes about sexual activity outside marriage has taken place. The media undoubtedly have contributed greatly to this.

Second, years ago fear of pregnancy used to be the chief reason young people abstained. Now birth control clinics offer confidential counseling to youth on how to use contraceptives.

But kids do not use contraceptives carefully. They also take chances, thinking first of all that they will be exempt—they won't get pregnant. And if it should happen to them, there will always be a way out. It is much the same as the one who smokes cigarettes, thinking others may get cancer but not he. Or the one who drives without a seat belt, thinking others will get injured in an accident but not she. Or the one who starts drinking alcoholic beverages—maybe even just beer—believing others will become alcoholics eventually but not she.

Making contraceptives and abortion readily available encourages risk-taking, and risk-taking leads to unwanted pregnancies.

18. *My dad says we shouldn't be deterred from having sex just because we're afraid of unwanted pregnancies. He says God's law forbids it, and that should be enough. I think that's legalism.*

I agree with your dad that as Christians we should not abstain from doing something just because we might be caught. We also shouldn't run risks and do forbidden things because we know of a way out if we are caught. I agree also that Christians surely should have regard for God's laws and His commandments. But I wonder if one of the reasons we pay so little attention to God's law is because we misunderstand it. We think of the law as a hammer held over our head. We don't view it as a hand held out in love to us.

---

[3]*Linacre Quarterly,* May 1982.

The Apostle Paul saw the law as an expression of love. "Love is the fulfilling of the law," he wrote (Rom. 13:10). Because we don't see the commandments as loving guidelines, intended to gift us with blessings, we haven't viewed them from a positive viewpoint. We haven't seen that they not only tell us what not to do, but they also show us how to do some very loving things. Martin Luther understood this positive function of the Ten Commandments. When the youth he was teaching asked him what the sixth commandment, "Thou shalt not commit adultery," meant, the answer he gave was, "We should fear and love God so that we lead a chaste and pure life in word and deed, and that husband and wife love and honor each other." That's positive!

Luther saw the sixth commandment against adultery as a gift of love to us from God. If we observe this commandment in a positive way, we shall enjoy a pure and healthy life, free from venereal disease. We shall be free from nagging doubts and guilt that come with premarital or extramarital sexual relationships. When we do finally marry, we will know how to love and honor each other if we follow this commandment of love. The fulfilling of the law, the obeying of God's commandments, becomes an act of love—love for God, for others and for ourselves.

19. *Are there any other books I could read on what to do if someone gets pregnant? I'd like to read more about abortion too.*

I can suggest two books. The first one is *Should I Keep My Baby?* by Martha Zimmerman.[4] This book discusses in detail the unwed mother's pregnancy and the options before her.

The second book, *Who Broke the Baby?*,[5] is by Jean Staker Garton. It is her own story, really. She used to aid the fight for easy availability of abortions, but as she continued to research the subject to gather support for her stance she experienced a complete change of conviction. "I spent many months of study and research examining the issue from various disciplines and perspectives," Dr. Garton writes. "I read the law, medicine and history. I studied Scripture and the church fathers. I worked long and hard to discover evidence to support my theory (of a mother's right of choice). But I found none."[6]

[4]Bethany House Publishers, 1983.
[5]Bethany House Publishers, 1979.
[6]Jean Staker Garton, *Who Broke the Baby?* (Minneapolis: Bethany House Publishers, 1979), p. 9.

Discussion of Abortion

(The resource book for this exercise is *Who Broke the Baby?* by Jean Staker Garton. The pages of her book that discuss the subjects introduced in this exercise are indicated in parentheses.)

1. In hotels thirteenth floors do not exist. Agree or disagree? (p. 14).
2. "Abortion is the first violence a child can experience at the hand of an adult." Agree or disagree? (p. 31).
3. Mothers should have the right to choose to abort a baby but fathers shouldn't. Agree or disagree? (p. 48).
4. Parents of a minor daughter should have the right to be involved in the abortion decision of their daughter. Agree or disagree?
5. "In the *Roe* v. *Wade* and *Doe* v. *Bolton* decisions of 1973, the Supreme Court provided examples of factors which would guide women in concluding that a child was unwanted and, therefore, 'abort-able': if the child might 'force upon the woman a distressful life or future' if she might be 'taxed by child care,' if she would experience 'embarrassment as a result of being unwed,' or if the birth of a child would 'deprive a woman of her preferred life style.' " With such criteria would God our heavenly Father have considered disowning and abandoning all of us? (p. 33).
6. What do the following phrases suggest to you, and why do you think pro-abortionists use them: termination of pregnancy; blob; mass of tissue; embryo; uterine contents; birth matter; the products of conception? Why do you think these terms instead of "person" or "baby" are used? (p. 37).
7. What do you think of this rationale: "I wouldn't enslave a black myself, but I support the right of others to choose to do so"? Compare that statement with: "I wouldn't have an abortion myself, but I give others the right to choose" (pp. 44, 45).
8. What do you understand by these phrases: "sex hang-up"; "neurotic inhibition"; "unhealthy repression"; "curative treatment"? What are these phrases meant to cover up? (pp. 87, 88).
9. Let us imagine you are married and you and your husband want to begin your family. If you could choose, would you choose to have a son or daughter? What do most people choose? As a result, what is happening? (p. 89).

10. Why does the statement "Every woman has a right to control her own body" still not give a woman the right to have an abortion? (p. 20 ff.).

Discussing the Use of Contraceptives

Discuss these questions with your parents:

1. If a married couple had intercourse regularly, and if the girl is 20 when she is married and experiences menopause (the cessation of her menstrual periods) when she is 46, how many children is it possible she could give birth to during the course of their married life?
2. Why may this not be desirable?
3. What factors affect the decision couples make as to how many children they will have?
4. What kind of people do you think should be encouraged to have more children than one or two?
5. What alternatives are there for increasing the size of one's family aside from giving birth to one's own children?

10 ❖ THE "LOVE BUG'S" DANGEROUS BITE

When we talk about reasons not to have sex outside of marriage, the most important consideration, of course, is that God has forbidden it. But some who are feeling rebellious won't care much about what God has to say on the matter. They might think a second or third time, though, if they realized the dangers to their health that lie in engaging in sex freely.

Diseases caught through sex are becoming more and more frequent. One of them, herpes, is impossible to cure. All of us need to know something about these diseases, how they are contracted, what they do to the body, and what the cures are, if there are any.

So we'll talk about that next.

Questions Kids Ask

1. *Does VD rash itch and burn?*

Syphilis rash does not itch or burn. With gonorrhea there is a severe burning sensation at the tip of the penis which may become swollen and inflamed. Most infected women, 85% to be exact, show no noticeable signs of having gonorrhea, which makes it very dangerous.

2. *Can you get VD even after you're married?*

If your spouse is infected, yes. Or if you have intercourse with someone else who has a disease, yes.

3. *Can you contract VD through oral sex?*
Yes, if the other person is infected.

4. *What do the initials STD stand for?*
"Sexually-transmitted diseases."

5. *Is it true necking causes skin diseases?*
Some venereal diseases can be contracted by kissing a person who has a sore on the lips or mouth. With syphilis a rash breaks out on the body in its second stage. Sometimes the rash is profuse. Sometimes it is so slight it is scarcely noticeable.

6. *I read about something called chlamydia. What is that?*
Chlamydia is the sexually-transmitted disease with the fastest rising incidence (three million to four million new cases last year). It can cause pelvic inflammatory disease which can fill the Fallopian tubes with scar tissue, increase the risk of a dangerous ectopic pregnancy and may make it impossible to have children. Chlamydia now ranks as a significant cause of infertility in women.

7. *Is VD as widespread as is claimed, or do people say it is just to scare kids?*
Genital herpes claimed 300,000 new victims in 1984. Venereal warts afflict 1 million new victims annually. AIDS doubled in incidence. Epidemiologists (experts on epidemics) estimate that about 27,000 new cases of sexually-transmitted diseases occur daily and that eventually, if the present trend continues, 25% of all Americans between the ages of 15 and 55 will be infected. Not only are the numbers frightening, but also the fact that many of the 25 known sexually-transmitted diseases have no known cure and last for a lifetime.

The effects of some of the diseases not only last a lifetime but may be passed on, with deadly consequences, to children of victims. For example, a mother who has active genital herpes may infect her baby during the process of birth. More than half of these infected infants die. Survivors are likely to have permanent brain damage. Some doctors try to perform Caesarean sections to save the babies, but in many cases it is not obvious that the mother is infected.

Chlamydia and venereal warts can also be passed on to newborn babies by their mothers. There have even been some cases in which infants caught AIDS from their mothers.

The epidemic is costly in dollars as well as lives. Already medical bills for treating sexually-transmitted diseases top $2 billion a year.

8. *Are VD or STD transferable only through intercourse?*
Venereal diseases are most commonly spread by intercourse

with an infected person, but they also can be contracted by kissing, or in rare occasions through a damp, infected towel; and cases have been reported of an STD being transmitted through a blood transfusion.

9. *Can you get drugs without a prescription to combat VD?*

No. The drugs used are antibiotics and must be prescribed by a doctor. If you have any doubts as to whether or not you are infected, see a doctor *right away*. Don't delay. Many forms of VD can be cured if you get help early enough.

10. *Can VD be contracted if no sperm are released?*

Yes. Contact with the genital parts of an infected person may be all that is needed to contract the disease.

11. *Someone said that kids who don't think they're worth much are most apt to get VD. Is this so?*

Studies have shown that in many cases those who contract VD have seen themselves as of little worth. Thinking themselves unlovable, victims of circumstances over which they have no control, they get depressed. So they try to find love and relief in any kind of sex relations available. The American media equate sex with love, so in their search for love and acceptance, these young people mistakenly turn to sex.

12. *What is the Wasserman test?*

The Wasserman test is used to identify syphilis.

Diseases Caught by Having Sex

Sexually-transmitted diseases or venereal diseases are very common and very dangerous. They are also very contagious, so you should know something about them. Test your knowledge by checking the true-false statements below. Answers are on the following page.

1. _____ More and more girls and women are developing genital infections because they have sex freely.

2. _____ In at least 15% of the cases, scar tissue in a woman's genital organs that prevents her from having babies is a result of having had gonorrhea at one time.

3. _____ Diseases such as gonorrhea and syphilis can be spread by oral sex.

4. _____ Pubic lice or "crabs" can be caught from sexual contact with someone who has them.

5. _____ Gonorrhea or "the clap" or "the drip," as some call it, can cause crippling arthritis.

6. _____ A man or boy has no way of knowing when he has caught gonorrhea.

7. _____ Usually a woman has no way of knowing she has contracted gonorrhea.

8. _____ Only men can transmit gonorrhea.

9. _____ Curing gonorrhea is possible.

10. _____ Gonorrhea can cause sterility in a man.

11. _____ Syphilis can kill.

12. _____ A mother who has syphilis can pass it on to her baby before her baby is born.

13. _____ It is easy to know when one has caught syphilis.

14. _____ If hair begins to fall out in patches, a person should check with a doctor.

15. _____ Syphilis usually burns itself out in a person's body.

16. _____ Venereal diseases can be caught by kissing.

17. _____ Venereal diseases can be caught from a toilet seat.

18. _____ If a boy or girl you do not know well presses you for sexual intercourse, be wary. The possibility exists that he or she may have one of the venereal diseases, or at least had it at one time.

19. _____ Herpes genitalis is caught by having sex with someone who has it.

20. _____ There is no cure for herpes.

21. _____ Pregnant women can pass on herpes to their unborn babies.

22. _____ Venereal diseases can be transmitted by oral sex.

Answers to Diseases Caught by Having Sex

1. *True.* These infections are known collectively as pelvic inflammatory diseases. These diseases cause scar tissue to develop in the Fallopian tubes, ovaries and uterus. Later, when a woman gets married and wants to have babies, this scar tissue can prevent her from having them.

2. *True.* In some cases the scar tissue is the result of another disease referred to as nonspecific urethritis, or NSU, or chlamydial infections. Many women who have this disease have no symptoms but pass on the disease when they have sex. If a man has symptoms, there will be painful urinating and a cloudy, mucous discharge from the penis. A woman also may feel the urge to urinate frequently and have a painful, burning sensation when she does so. Anyone having these symptoms should check with a doctor.

It is possible to have a urinary infection caused by bacteria that have no relationship to sexual diseases. So if you have trouble urinating, don't be afraid to tell your parents just because you think they will accuse you of having been promiscuous, when you haven't. In any case, if you have symptoms, see a doctor.

3. *True.* (See answer for 22.)

4. *True.* Pubic lice are blood-sucking lice that usually appear in the pubic hair and the hair around the anus. Normal washing will not remove either them or the eggs the females lay. It may take several weeks to find out you have pubic lice because it takes them time to breed. The only symptom may be itching, particularly at night. A doctor can give you a lotion to shampoo to kill the lice and eggs.

5. *True.* Gonorrhea, if not treated properly, can cause crippling arthritis and sterility.

6. *False.* It is very easy for a man to know when he has gonorrhea, but he must pay attention to the first symptoms. When he urinates, it will burn painfully. Pus will also drip from his penis.

7. *True.* It is very difficult for a woman to know if she has contracted gonorrhea. Therefore if a man or a boy discovers he has it, he should get in contact with any girl or girls with whom he has had intercourse so they can have an examination. If the girl's gonorrhea is not treated, it will damage her body.

8. *False.* Women who have gonorrhea can transmit it to

men through sexual intercourse.

9. *True.* Penicillin or other antibiotics are very effective. But these antibiotics do not provide immunity.

10. *True.* If not treated, gonorrhea attacks the joints and sex organs. When the body tries to repair the damage, scar tissue may form which may block the sperm in a man or the egg in a woman, preventing them from escaping.

11. *True.* Syphilis has the power to kill if it is not treated properly. Years ago thousands died because of syphilis. With the antibiotics available now, it is not necessary for any to die because of syphilis.

12. *True.* There are at least a quarter million new cases of syphilis a year in the U.S. A pregnant woman should always be tested for the disease.

13. *False.* Syphilis appears first as a hard, painless, moist sore on a man's penis or deep in a woman's vagina where she may not be aware of it at all. The sore can appear anytime from a few days to a month after a person has contracted it through sexual intercourse. If a person does not pay attention to this sore or isn't aware of it, the disease will go "underground," and the damage will be serious. The sore is called a chancre (pronounced "shanker") and is red and solid and protrudes above the skin. These sores can appear elsewhere on the body too, frequently on the mouth or rectum.

14. *True.* Hair falling out in patches is one of the symptoms of syphilis. A nonitching rash on the palms or soles of feet is another. The person may also have a sore throat, low fever and aching limbs.

15. *False.* The symptoms disappear, but the disease burrows itself deeper into the body and begins to cause massive problems, even death.

16. *True.* If one has a chancre (sore) or syphilitic patches in the mouth, then the disease can be transmitted by "deep kissing."

17. *False.* The chances that venereal diseases will be caught from toilet seats are slim because the germs can stay alive only a few minutes if they do not remain moist and remain at body temperature. Because of this they can't live long on doorknobs either. But it's still wise for people to take precautions against wet toilet seats. (Besides, who enjoys sitting on a wet toilet seat?)

18. *True.* Usually people who have intercourse with many partners have the disease.

19. *True.* With herpes, groups of blisters develop on one or several areas. The blisters rupture and become shallow ulcers or sores. About six days after contact with an infected person you may feel pain, tenderness or an itchy sensation near the penis or vulva. You may also run a fever, have a headache or just generally feel ill. The blisters appear along a man's penis or a woman's vulva, but also may occur on the thighs or buttocks. In a woman, if the blisters form only inside the vagina, she has no way of knowing she has the disease and may pass it on to others without knowing she has done so.

When the blisters break, they form open sores of raw, exposed skin or ulcers. This is very, very painful. The ulcers last from one to three weeks. After the blisters subside, recurrences may take place in the months or years following. A doctor may prescribe soothing ointments or frequent warm baths to reduce the pain, but there is little else that can be done.

In addition, if herpes invades people who are having problems with kidney, lung or blood diseases, their condition becomes worse.

20. *True.* A drug called Isoprinosine is producing some results in relieving the effects of herpes, but it is not a cure.

21. *True.* If the patient has an active case of herpes at the time of labor and delivery she can pass on the disease to her child.

22. *True.* Venereal diseases can be caught from oral sex. Young people who are resorting to oral sex because they want to have sex but want to avoid pregnancies should know this very real danger exists.

Chilling facts, aren't these? Don't you wonder why anyone ever risks having sex outside of marriage?

Where can a young person turn for help if he thinks he has one of these diseases and is afraid to tell his parents? He can call National VD Hotline (1–800–227–8922, or in California 1–800–982–5883). Or call your family doctor or go to a health clinic. Look in your telephone directory under the name of city, county, or state and then "Health Department."

Another place to turn to is a church. There you should also be able to find love, a listening ear, help and also the right kind of friends.

11 ❖ QUESTIONS AND ANSWERS ON TOUGH SUBJECTS

Masturbation

1. *What does masturbation mean?*

Masturbation is the name for producing pleasurable, sexual feelings or sensations by rubbing genital parts against each other or by stroking or caressing one's own breasts, thighs, or genital parts. It is a feeling similar to what people experience when they have intercourse. Sometimes the stimulation is continued until orgasm is experienced.

Because this is a subject that has differing viewpoints among Christians and because the Bible does not make a direct statement either for or against it, you no doubt will want to hear your parents' and your pastor's ideas on it along with the facts in this chapter.

2. *I was just sitting studying for an exam and got all restless because I'd been sitting so long, and suddenly I started to get all sorts of excited feelings. The more I moved, the more excited I got, and my penis got erect and finally semen came out and then I felt all relaxed and at peace, and yet I was embarrassed. What happened? Should this not have happened?*

The experience you describe is one of the ways young people sometimes masturbate without being aware that they are doing so. In your adolescent years certain areas of your body become keenly responsive to touch. Touching arouses sexual sensations. Even just walking or running can produce these feelings.

These feelings are a very normal experience and nothing to be ashamed about.

3. *Will weird things happen to me if I masturbate?*
All doctors agree that masturbation will cause no physical harm or problems.

Many kids masturbate at some time or other. Some masturbation seems to be almost a spontaneous natural response to the strong sexual urges and drives a young person feels. Sometimes it's sort of like an exploration to find out which parts of the body cause excitement and strange, enjoyable feelings.

But a word of warning is in order here: Even though the Bible makes no direct statement about masturbation, the Bible has a great deal to say about lust and impure thoughts. As Dr. William Backus has noted: "Almost surely, the reason why Christians have cautioned against masturbation is that masturbation is normally accompanied by fantasies of sexual activity. If what is fantasized is deviant and sinful, then the behavior is lust. And lust is clearly forbidden by Jesus."[1] Dr. Backus also believes that masturbation can shape sexual responses, including sexual deviation.

Our sexual organs were designed for *giving*, for expressing love to one's spouse. Therefore, many Christians believe that to masturbate is to misuse God's gift for our own pleasure, and such selfishness which defrauds one's spouse would violate God's pattern of sacrificial, other-centered love.

4. *My boyfriend knows I don't believe in intercourse now, but he wants me to rub his thighs and penis. I don't feel good about this, but when I tell him this, he says I don't really love him because I'm not willing to satisfy his needs. Would it be wrong for me to do what he wants me to do?*
Masturbating in the sense of touching the genital parts of another person almost always leads to intercourse. It's like trying to drive on a freeway without ever having learned how to drive a car and expecting that you won't get into an accident.

Sorry. Such mutual stimulation is for married people. So stay clear of any petting below the neck.

And don't let your boyfriend intimidate you by threatening you. True love never intimidates or threatens. Don't be afraid

---

[1]William Backus, *Telling the Truth to Troubled People* (Minneapolis: Bethany House Publishers, 1985), p. 242.

to stand up for what you believe. In the end people will respect you for it.

5. *Do girls play with themselves or masturbate as often as boys do?*
No. Boys masturbate more.

6. *Are you abnormal if you don't ever masturbate?*
Of course not. Many young people, because they simply are not so inclined or, because of Christian and moral convictions, never consciously masturbate.

Homosexuality

1. *What is meant by homosexual behavior?*
Homosexual behavior is physical, sexual contact between two persons of the same gender, between two men or two women, a contact that usually results in sexual arousal. People who are homosexual in their response desire physical contact with someone of their own gender: Thinking about or seeing someone of their own gender who is attractive to them can arouse them sexually.

2. *I'm afraid I have a crush on one of my teachers. The problem is I'm a girl and she's a woman. Does the fact that I like her so much mean I'm turning into a homosexual?*
Not at all. It's not uncommon for teen-age girls to be drawn to women and boys to men. Perhaps one of the reasons for this is adolescents are trying to break free from their mothers and fathers in order to achieve independence. At the same time they are not feeling very secure. Consequently they find an older friend, a man or a woman, who for the time being takes the place of their parents as far as offering support, love and encouragement, but at the same time allows the young person to achieve a measure of independence.

3. *I have a friend whom I love very much. We share the same interests, and we enjoy each other. But we are both fellows. Being we're so close to each other, is there danger we'll become homosexuals?*
The Bible gives many examples of people of the same sex who were as close to each other as the thumb is to the thumbnail. Think of David and Jonathan (1 Sam. 18:1–4; 20:17, 23,

40–42; 2 Sam. 1:26). David loved Jonathan "as he loved himself," and Jonathan loved David. They covenanted to be friends forever. They asked the Lord to bless their friendship. When they had to say good-bye to each other for a while, they would cry and hug each other. But there is no indication that they were homosexual.

Or consider the close relationship between Paul and the younger Timothy. Or even more astonishing, between Ruth and her mother-in-law, Naomi.

It is also possible for a woman to have a man as a close friend and yet have nothing sexual in the relationship. Jesus evidently felt close to Mary and Martha and often visited them.

In all of these friendships there was no sexual relationship. Instead, love in its truest form is what binds the two together. So enjoy your friend. Accept him as a gift from God.

4. *Some of the guys at school want to touch me when I go to the bathroom—I mean touch me in places I don't want to be touched by them. Are they homosexuals? What can I do?*

They may not be homosexuals. Some boys think it's smart to masturbate each other. Some just try to humiliate and embarrass others.

But what to do? That can be a real problem. I've known kids who haven't dared to drink liquids all day because they didn't want to go to the toilet, either for the reason you give, or because of marijuana or cigarette smoke being so strong in the biffy. That's rough. If you have a teacher whom you can trust and talk with, maybe you can get permission to go during a class period when the bathroom is more apt to be empty. And have you discussed your problem with your parents?

5. *Are some people born homosexuals?*

Dr. William Backus, a Christian psychologist in St. Paul, Minnesota, in *Telling the Truth to Troubled People*, states that many psychologists believe homosexual behavior is learned. If a person is normal physically and mentally, he says there is no evidence that there are any hormonal, chromosomal or organic differences between a homosexual person and a heterosexual person.[2]

Homosexuality is not new. During the era of the Greek empire, it was practiced as a form of birth control. Families at that

---

[2]Backus, pp. 244–247.

time tried to limit the number of children to two, three at the most—possibly a second son in case one son died. In order to limit the size of the families, houses were built with separate quarters for men and women. The husband was allowed to visit his wife's bedroom only at certain times. To satisfy his sexual hungers in between he kept boys who had been trained in the art of homosexuality. Sometimes this training was given in the gymnasia. At the entrance to many gymnasia an idol of the god of homosexuality would be found, and he was worshiped by the young boys of the gymnasia. Homosexuality for the Greeks at that time definitely was a learned response.

6. *My dad says masturbating can turn fellows into homosexuals. How can that be?*

Let's think first about how habits are formed. Let's say a person is worried—extremely worried. A friend gives him a tranquilizer. His feelings of anxiety disappear. He feels calm and relaxed and at peace. It's a good feeling. Next time he gets worried, he asks his friend for a tranquilizer. The more he uses them, the more he wants them. If something gives him pleasure or makes him feel good, chances are he'll want to turn to it more and more.

Now let's suppose a neighbor whom a young boy likes and trusts begins to fondle the boy. The boy finds the feelings pleasurable.

"That's neat!" he says.

"I'll teach you how to do it," says the man. "Then you can do it to me, and I can do it to you, and you can do it by yourself too."

The boy is delighted. He feels grown up. He begins to masturbate by himself more and more. As he does, he thinks of his "friend" and sometimes imagines he's with him. He feels closer and closer to him. Finally he discovers he's more comfortable with men than with women. The pattern he has been following has become a habit.

7. *Can homosexuals change?*

If they want to, yes. The Apostle Paul referred to some in the Christian congregation at Corinth who had changed. "Do you not know that the wicked will not inherit the kingdom of God? Do not be deceived: Neither the sexually immoral nor idolaters nor adulterers nor male prostitutes nor homosexual offenders nor thieves nor the greedy nor drunkards nor slanderers nor swindlers will inherit the kingdom of God. *And that is what some of you were.* But you were washed, you were sanctified, you were justified in the name of the Lord Jesus Christ and by the Spirit of our God" (1 Cor. 6:9–11, NIV).

Also *The American Journal of Psychiatry*, in its December 1980, issue, published an article documenting change in eleven men who once were homosexuals but who changed after becoming Christians.

But a homosexual must *want* to change and must be willing to cooperate with God in this process. The trouble is that most homosexuals are so satisfied and contented with their lives that they don't want to change. God never forces himself upon a person. A person must be willing to change if he is to experience God's help.

8. *Can a homosexual change suddenly?*

If homosexuality is a learned behavior, learned over a period of time, then it follows that to unlearn it will usually take time. It is a process.

The first step is to get the person's beliefs changed. Usually we act according to what we believe. Dr. Backus, in his book, lists many misbeliefs homosexuals have. If a homosexual is going to change, he first must change these misbeliefs, and in their place accept scriptural truths. Below is a list of a few of these misbeliefs. You probably have heard some of them. As an exercise, underneath each statement, write what the Bible teaches.

- "What feels good is good."

- "Everybody else has a glorious, free sex life, doing exactly as he wishes. It's unfair if I can't do the same."

- "Homosexuals who are faithful to their partners are just the same as heterosexuals who are faithful to theirs."

- "It's bad for me not to express whatever sexual desires I happen to feel. I'll get neurotic if I don't."

- "If I can't, for a time, engage in any sex at all, I'll have to be absolutely miserable."

- "I am not responsible for my behavior. I *have* to do it. I couldn't stand *not* doing it. Someone else *makes* me do it."

- "There should be a magic miraculous instant cure for my deviant sexual urges or I have no reason to be interested in change."

- "If God wants me different, He should make me different."[3]

It should be noted that in addition to changing beliefs, the homosexual person wanting to change may need the skilled help of a professional counselor. Many churches have counselors on their staffs or can refer people to Christian counselors.

9. *Aren't sexual sins the worst sins of all?*

Sin is sin. Sin, regardless which sin it is, separates us from God. That's what makes sin so serious. Some sinful acts may be termed "worse" than others because they affect other people—that is, others suffer because of our sinning. But if the Holy Spirit has shown us what our hearts are like apart from God, we'll neither look down on anyone nor be surprised by anything a person does. We know that we are capable of doing the same.

10. *Can a person be involved in sexual sins and still be a Christian?*

Let's ask this question: Can a person be involved in any sin and be a Christian? The answer, of course, is that Christians, not being perfect, may sin from time to time, whether it be in wrong sexual relationships, or in not forgiving someone, or in cheating or neglecting to show love, or whatever. The question to ask is: Does this person consciously and willfully continue to do this sinful act, or does he want to, and does he cooperate with the Holy Spirit, to be freed? Christians will be tempted even as other people are tempted. What should make a Christian different is the way he responds to temptation.

11. *Can women be homosexuals too?*

Yes, they are called lesbians.

12. *Can a homosexual be married and have children?*

Yes, but sooner or later almost unbearable tensions develop, so such marriages often break up.

13. *I'm interested in a career, but it scares me because I've heard*

---

[3]Backus, pp. 250, 251.

it said that a typical career woman has hidden lesbian tendencies.

That is completely false. Most career women are happy, well-adjusted heterosexual women. Many are married and have families. Today it is possible to have both a good marriage and a satisfying career, though it does call for careful planning and discipline.

14. *Would a man who feels your penis be homosexual?*

Not necessarily. He could be a man occupied with masturbating other boys and men. Nonetheless, I'd say: "Hands off my private property!"

Child Abuse

1. *Who abuses kids? Strangers who catch you on the street?*

No. Sexual child abuse is committed most often by someone the child knows: a relative, friend or neighbor. In cases of incest, in more than half the cases the offender is the stepfather.

2. *What can a kid do to prevent being abused?*

Learn that it's all right to say no to an adult. If you feel uncomfortable the way an adult hugs or kisses you, resist, push the adult away, and if necessary, yell or run away.

3. *What should a girl do if the man in the home where she is baby-sitting comes back home and begins to play around with her?*

If he abuses you in any way, tell someone. Don't keep secrets from your parents. If it does happen to you, remember it isn't your fault. Find someone with whom you can talk and talk. Get everything out of your mind that is troubling you. Ask God to heal your memories and help you forgive the one who has wronged you.

4. *Why don't kids tell?*

Often they are threatened, so they are afraid to tell. Some don't want anything bad to happen to the one who has molested them. Most kids have mixed-up feelings. They want to tell and they don't want to. Some feel ashamed.

5. *When a man offers you money to let him fool around, what does he actually want to do?*

He wants to have sex with you in one way or another and play around with you sexually as he pleases. Don't ever risk it!

Oral Sex

1. *I've heard the kids at school talking about oral sex, but I guess I'm dumb—I don't know what it is. And I'm embarrassed to ask. Can you explain?*

The word "oral" means "mouth." Oral sex is using the mouth to stimulate the partner's sex organs.

2. *Some of the kids at school are practicing oral sex. They say, what's wrong about it? Isn't it better than a girl getting pregnant? And it isn't intercourse, so what's wrong with it? I still don't feel good about it though, but I don't know how to answer them.*

First of all, oral sex cannot be practiced without a girl and boy revealing their bodies to each other. There is something special and beautiful about waiting to unveil our body to our one true love after the wedding. To unveil my body to a number of others cheapens the gift that is mine to give. It becomes a pawed-over, shop-worn gift. Shouldn't we want the gift of our body to be a gift saved for our husband or wife?

But even more serious than the unveiling of our bodies to those whom we do not intend to marry is the fact that oral sex is engaged in to produce orgasm. What difference is there then between oral sex and intercourse, aside from the fact that pregnancy is not risked? Oral sex is just another form of fornication when unmarried people engage in it. The Bible is very straightforward about declaring fornication to be sin. Look up these verses: Mark 7:21; 1 Corinthians 6:13–20; Galatians 5:19ff.; Ephesians 5:3ff.; 1 Thessalonians 4:1–8; Hebrews 13:4; Revelation 2:20.

Young people need to know also that venereal diseases can be transmitted by oral sex.

Other Tough Subjects

1. *Why do men rape women?*

In most cases rape is a crime of violence and rage. Men usually rape, not because they are attracted sexually to a person, but because they are angry and want to hurt people. That's why they will attack even old women. Women who are raped need feel no sense of shame or guilt and should report the crime immediately. And if you ever are attacked, never, never hesitate to tell your parents immediately. Also, because rape is a crime of violence, it's best not to resist if the one attacking is armed in any way.

2. *What is a transvestite?*

The transvestite is a man who likes to wear women's clothing, either one piece such as a bra or a whole outfit complete with makeup. Transvestites usually don't like their bodies and disown their maleness. They want to live the life of a woman and have sexual relations with a man in the same way a woman would. So they are different from homosexuals.

Some transvestites go so far as to take hormone therapy that will cause their breasts to develop, their voice to become more like a woman's and their whiskers to become sparse and soft. A few even have their penis and testicles removed surgically and have an artificial vagina fashioned.

3. *I read about women going to doctors to have sperm put into them. What's that all about?*

The doctor collects sperm from the husband and puts it in the wife's vagina with an instrument. If the sperm finds an egg in the woman, the woman will get pregnant. Some couples who haven't been able to get pregnant in the usual way try this method. It is referred to as artificial insemination.

4. *Do some babies grow in test tubes, or what is meant by test tube babies?*

Doctors take sperm from the husband and an egg from the mother and put them together in a container. If a sperm and egg unite, this embryo is placed inside the mother's uterus with an instrument, and the baby grows inside the mother as usual. Sometimes this works, sometimes it doesn't.

5. *I thought only young girls had to be concerned about being raped, but I read about an old woman being raped. How could she be attractive to a young man?*

It has been found that, typically, the rape victim is between 18 and 25, although young children and old women are not immune.

The rapist, typically, although there are always exceptions, is about 26, from a low-income, culturally-deprived background. Sometimes he is mentally retarded or of low intelligence. Often he has emotionally unstable parents and sometimes an alcoholic father. Most rapists come from broken homes and have grown up with little discipline. They are used to taking what they want, whether it be money, a car, or a woman. That is why, most often, rape is a crime of violence.

6. *Is there any connection with pornographic pictures and the bad way people sometimes act?*

The U.S. Justice Department is studying the relationship between pornography and wrong sexual behavior. But Franciscan priest Bruce Ritter, who gives sanctuary to abused children in his Covenant House in New York, believes there is a direct connection. "The most intellectually dishonest thing a person can say," he asserts, "is that there is no connection between pornography and sexual abuse and deviations."

Suzanne Danielson, who handles child abuse cases for the state of Louisiana, believes that a child's resistance is broken down when he is shown pornographic pictures. If a child sees something in a magazine, she says, the child begins to believe it must be all right.

7. *I've heard it said that people who rape or abuse kids are oversexed and can't help themselves. Is this true?*

No. They simply turn their sex impulses in the wrong direction and misuse them.

12 ❖ HOW CAN I TALK WITH MY PARENTS ABOUT THESE THINGS?

Growing up isn't easy, is it? Maybe you feel unprepared for the future. Or you worry about school or about not being popular. If you're a girl, you maybe worry about sexual attacks on the streets.

Many of you already have formed values, good values, but you wonder if you'll be able to stay true to your convictions. Some of you worry about death. Some of you wonder if you will amount to anything in life. And some of you still have questions about sex. And if you've gone through this book on your own, you wish you could talk to your parents about some of these things. "Why are parents so embarrassed to talk about sex?" you ask.

I can't really answer for your parents, but I can guess at some of the reasons. Not too long ago in our society, people didn't talk about sex freely. Some thought it was "dirty." Some thought it was a private matter. Maybe your grandparents never talked to your parents about sex. Maybe your parents have never gotten used to talking about sex. Maybe they think talking about sex means talking about *their* sex life, and they want to keep that private (which is right). Maybe they don't have the proper information, and so they're afraid you'll ask questions they can't answer. Whatever the reason, they're hesitant.

What can you do?

You can try saying, "Mom and Dad, I have some questions that are very important to me. You might feel a little embarrassed when you hear them, just as I'm a little embarrassed to ask them, but I'd really rather talk with you about them than with anybody else."

Another thing you can do is to work at developing a better relationship with your parents. Instead of yelling at them or throwing things or walking off in a huff when they correct you, try saying something like this: "I get it. You don't like it when I play my stereo so loud," or, "Oh, I see. You wish I'd keep my room in better order."

If you possibly can bring yourself to go on to say, "I'm sorry. I'll really try to do better," you'll melt your parents' hearts. If you add a hug to that, *Wow!*

If you think your parents' criticism is unfair and they have misunderstood, tell them so in a quiet, respectful tone. Chances are good that they will respect you. Say, "Sorry," and negotiate.

Try hard not to give the impression that you know it all. If you run into a situation in which you think you *do* understand better than your parents do (such as, what to wear), you may tell them so, but again, respectfully.

And why not try going one step further? Have you ever thought of getting your parents to talk about themselves, their feelings, their worries, their experiences, etc., and then listening to them? Here are some questions that could serve as openers.

What do you worry about?

What makes you happy?

If you could have three wishes, what would they be?

How do you feel at the end of a workday?

How do you feel when you wake up?

When you think of us kids, what do you wish for us? Fear for us?

Do you really like your job?

If you could live any place in the world, where would you like to live?

If you were a teen-ager starting your life over, would you do anything different?

What would you like to change in our family?

What do you like the most about our family?

You shouldn't ask all these questions at one time. Rather, slip in one question at a time when you can. I promise you'll find out things about your parents you never knew before, and you'll begin to understand them better. And if you can get them talking about these things, chances are it will be easier to talk with them about things that are on your heart too. It's worth a try—not just a halfhearted, I'll-try-it-once try, but a patient, day-after-day try.

One thing more. How about a little old-fashioned courtesy toward your parents: "Thank you." "Please." "That was a supergood meal, Mom!" "I like the way you barbecue chicken, Dad!" "You look tired. May I finish the vacuuming?" "I can unload the dishwasher tonight." "If spaghetti is all right, I can make supper."

You've no idea what that will do for your parents! All along they've thought you were the best kids any parents could ever have. Now they *know* it.

All of this we've written about is what love is really about. As the Apostle Paul explained: "Love is patient, love is kind. It does not envy, it does not boast, it is not proud. It is not rude, it is not self-seeking, it is not easily angered, it keeps no record of wrongs. Love does not delight in evil but rejoices with the truth. It always protects, always trusts, always hopes, always perseveres. Love never fails" (1 Cor. 13:4–8, NIV).

And when your time finally comes either to walk down the aisle or to stand up front and greet the one walking down the aisle toward you, you'll discover for yourself that it is this love that makes sexual love so super wonderful, and home such a happy, secure place.

Happy future, young friend! God go with you.

13 ❖ YEARS LATER . . .

Meghan at Twenty-five

I don't know why, God, but here on the beach I can think. The breakers washing in, the sea gulls dipping and soaring overhead, the rain-laden dark clouds moving up from the horizon, the wind whipping my hair, the salty mist stinging my face—all help to clear my troubled mind.

Sometimes, Father, I feel overwhelmed because life seems so complex. Demand after demand is pushing its way into my life. But absorbed as I am in the lives of others, something deep within me never lets me forget that I am also an individual, a unique being endowed by God with certain distinctive abilities, given to me that I might contribute in some small way to the happiness and welfare of others.

I also am—and I never cease to wonder at it—your child, Father. I thank you that the sacrifice of your Son made this relationship possible. This relationship brings life into focus for me, lifts me out of despair, puts courage in my heart, and gives me the faith to believe that in the end, all will be well.

You know the concern that nags me so much of the time, loving Father, as to when I'll meet the man to whom I joyfully can join my life. Sometimes I become anxious, wondering if maybe I never will get married. I wonder if I could handle that. But you will care for me in this regard too, won't you, dear God? In the quietness of this hour reassure me.

From time to time I also struggle with feeling really good about my body, Lord. I wish I had a nicer figure. But it is getting easier to accept my body's shape. As I try to discipline myself and care for my body, help me not to dwell on this aspect of my life. Instead, help me to forget myself, to become absorbed in reaching out.

For when I turn my back to the sea and face the city, where the evening lights are beginning to twinkle, I think of all those back there in the city who need you. The smug, self-satisfied ones who don't feel a need of you. The frustrated, angry ones. The lonely ones. Those who are constantly downgraded. The children of broken homes. The confused students in schools and universities. The homesick overseas students. The forgotten old people. The minority groups. I care, Father, I do. But though my heart weeps with you, that so many thousands are estranged from you, yet I thank you that you are their Savior, that you love and care.

But caring is not enough. I need to hear your voice so I can understand what you want me, as an individual, to do. I can't do it all. But with your enabling, I can do what you ask me to do. That's why I'm walking the beach tonight, Father. Speak to me. Make clear to me your will.

Then I know I shall go walking through the days ahead, confident of my calling, assured of your leading, strong in your provision, exulting in my privilege, and serene in my hope and expectation.

Peter at Twenty-five

I can't sleep tonight. Tomorrow Kathy and I will join our lives together. Awe and wonder sweep over me, dear God, as I think of the gracious gift you are giving me in Kathy. Has a young man ever found such a sweet, loving, understanding, gentle young woman as I have? I don't deserve her, but I do thank you, dear God, for her.

You have been so faithful and good to me. The teen years were so difficult. First, there was the agony of the bad case of acne that plagued me. My doctor said it was one of the worst he had seen. We tried everything, but nothing seemed to help. I suffered every time I looked in the mirror.

Then along came petite, pretty Ruthie, who didn't seem to see my acne. We clicked immediately. Two gloriously happy years followed.

Because of the medication I couldn't be out in the sun. That ruled out beach parties with the gang. It also meant no more baseball or tennis in the summer. And with my back so full of eruptions I couldn't bear the thought of going on a basketball floor again. But Ruthie didn't seem to mind. We found things to do together, just the two of us, when I couldn't go along with the others.

And then suddenly my world crumbled about me when Ruthie told me one day that she had found someone she loved more than me. I couldn't believe it! The anger I had felt when the acne wouldn't clear up, and the resentment that had simmered when I had had to give up sports burst into a roaring flame of rage. You remember how it was, Jesus. Alone in my room, door locked, I stormed and fumed. I pounded the bed with my fists. To lose the one girl who had seemed to love me simply for who I was seemed just too much.

I still think what a miracle it was the way you met me those days. Alone in my room one night we had it out between the two of us. Tearfully I was able finally to turn myself over to you, to say that I would trust you whatever, that you and doing your will was more important to me than anything else. You met me at that point. I can still remember the relief that came when I felt the load I had been carrying slide off. I felt light and happy. Peace flooded my heart. The change was so fantastic I couldn't believe it.

The next day—remember?—I got an award for being the outstanding bowler of our class. If I had received that award earlier, all my former ambitions to excel in sports would have grabbed hold of me. But as it was, though I was glad for my trophy, it did not control me. You, Jesus, were in control of my life.

And then you brought Kathy to my side. Dear, dear Kathy. I was so glad when I met her that Ruthie and I, though we'd been close friends, had never "gone the whole way."

At the same time you began to give me a sense of direction for my life. More years of graduate schooling still stretch ahead of me. But Kathy has assured me of her loyal support. I want to see her happy too, Lord. I want to see her develop and use to the full the talents and abilities you have given her.

As I lie here, this last night I'll spend as an unmarried son in my parents' home, I want to thank you for them too, dear God, for their love and support. Thank you that we are so close to each other. Thank you for all the good times we've had together.

Thank you, too, for Kathy's parents. I'm so glad that our families have the same values.

I wonder what the years ahead will hold and where you will

lead us. I wonder how many children we'll have and what they will be like. Somehow I can't be worried about the future tonight. Your presence with me here by the side of my bed is so real to me, Jesus. I feel as though I could almost reach out and touch you. With you to hold our hands, what do we have to fear?

Take our lives, Jesus. May they be spilled out in love for you and for others who need you. To walk with you and do your will is such *joy*! Thank you, Jesus. Thank you.